HOW TO LIVE TO 90

HOW TO LIVE TO 90

(with a bit of luck)

James Le Fanu

Robinson
London
IN COLLABORATION WITH THE DAILY TELEGRAPH

Constable & Robinson Ltd
3 The Lanchesters
162 Fulham Palace Road
London W6 9ER

First published in 1991 by Papermac, as *Health Wise*

This revised edition published by Robinson, an imprint of
Constable & Robinson Ltd 2000

A copy of the British Library Cataloguing in Publication
data is available from the British Library

ISBN 1–84119–102–7

Printed and bound in the EC

CONTENTS

INTRODUCTION

The Queen dispatches nearly 2000 telegrams a year to centenarians compared to a mere 200 when she first ascended the throne – testimony indeed to the astonishing increase in longevity that has occurred during the almost fifty years of her reign. The centenarian remains a rare bird, but the average lifespan for both sexes has risen well into the eighties, so the ambition to 'get to ninety' is not unreasonable – but how to do it? My inspiration for writing this book came just before my own fiftieth birthday. Like most people I had been blessed with rudely good health for my first four decades, rarely bothering to consult the doctor except for the occasional nasty bout of flu. Then two things happened in quick succession. First, I noticed while getting into the bath that the water around my left leg was much cooler than that around the right. Despite turning on the hot tap again and swishing the water around, the curious sensation persisted, at which point I realised the problem was not the temperature of the bath, rather that my left leg was no longer able to perceive heat. I was naturally rather alarmed as to what could be the cause of this unusual symptom so made an urgent medical appointment. My doctor referred me to a neurologist to sort out the leg problem and for good measure took my blood pressure, which turned out to be sufficiently raised to warrant treatment.

So within a few days I had moved from being apparently healthy and carefree to having two medical problems – both of which might if left untreated have had quite serious consequences. This naturally changed my perception of the future and I started to have, as many before me, intimations of mortality. It seemed that I clearly had to take steps to maximise my chances of living longer if I were still to fulfil my ambitions and watch my children grow to maturity.

The most important determinant of a long life are the genes inherited from one's parents – longevity runs very strongly in families – nonetheless the steady increase in lifespan over the last century shows there are other more modifiable factors as well. Some of these are obvious and commonsensical, such as not smoking and making efforts to stay fit with regular exercise. But other elements involved in 'living longer' have only become apparent in recent years, particularly the development of screening techniques to detect cancer early and the use of preventive drugs like aspirin to keep the blood flowing. As, surprisingly, there is no popular accessible account of current knowledge on these matters, it seemed only sensible to change my reflections on 'how to get to ninety' into this book. So, what are its main themes?

First, from the fifties onwards people become vulnerable to 'sniper fire' from one or other of three major illnesses: cancer, heart disease and stroke. Some, but by no means all, of these sniper fire casualties can be avoided, thus permitting an extra decade of life or more. Most people would think this well worthwhile.

Second, there is more to 'getting to ninety' than staying alive, as the autumn years should also be as pleasurable as possible and we should all hope to be healthy enough to enjoy them. Chronologically we may get older, but 'our inner selves' do not age and we need to know how, as far as possible, we can maintain our youthful vigour by keeping the skeleton strong, the heart pumping vigorously and the brain ticking over.

This book seeks to clarify these important matters but will also, I hope, serve a third purpose. If we become a trifle fearful about the future once the wrong side of fifty, it is mainly because we cannot imagine what problems we may encounter. There are, after all, so many things that can go wrong and so much contradictory advice about what we should and should not be doing. The crucial fact that most people remain remarkably healthy can too readily be obscured by an over-active imagination about hidden but non-existent dangers. So this book will, I hope, also provide a sense of perspective within which the future can be approached with an appropriate degree of equanimity.

We start with The Big Picture, which explains in simple terms what happens as we get older. Then we turn to those topics already alluded to in which guidance can be helpful. In Part 1 Living Longer, we consider how a 'healthy' lifestyle, screening and preventive drugs can keep us robust and protect us against the Big Three snipers – cancer, heart disease and strokes. In the next section, When Things Go Wrong, we learn of the sort of medical problems that do occur and how best they can be resolved. This falls readily into three self explanatory sections, Is It Serious?, Sorting Things Out and Putting Things Right. Part 3 considers the many ways in which it is possible to minimise the physical changes of ageing, so we can 'Stay Beautiful, Perceptive, Mobile, Cheerful and Sexy'. Finally, 'Battling the Big Three' discusses current medical approaches to the treatment of heart attacks, strokes and cancer.

THE BIG PICTURE

The most dynamic process in the human body is the ability of cells to renew themselves by dividing to form 'new' cells. In this way, and it is an extraordinary if underappreciated fact, our faces, for example, are literally 'replaced' every eighteen months. The cells divide to form a new layer of skin, while just beneath the same process renews the connective tissue and elastic fibres, keeping the surface of the skin smooth. There is, however, a limit to this facility of replication – the 'Hayflick' limit – named after the scientist who first identified it in the early 1960s. A single cell, having divided and renewed itself forty-six times (or thereabouts) divides no more. The changes in facial appearance once this limit is reached are only too familiar – wrinkles, crow's feet and dropping of the cheeks and neck.

In a similar way, the Hayflick limit means that the functions of various organs and tissues of the body will decline over time: the speed with which electrical impulses travel down the nerves, the amount of blood pumped out by the heart, the blood flow through the kidneys and the amount of air the lungs can exhale all fall to about half their youthful capacity.

None of these changes is as serious as they might sound and for two reasons. Firstly, the functional reserve of our kidneys, hearts and lungs is considerable, so despite the decline with age, there is more than enough capacity to see out the last decades of life. Secondly, many of the adverse effects of ageing are readily amenable to medical or surgical treatment. Wrinkles and drooping jaws can be corrected with plastic surgery, a lens implant will reverse the loss of vision due to clouded cataracts, a plastic joint restores mobility to arthritic hips and an operation on the prostate will restore urine flow.

It is not possible to be quite so optimistic about the Big Three 'snipers': heart disease, strokes and cancer. These, too, are 'age related' – that is, the likelihood of suffering from one or the other rises with each passing decade. They represent, as already pointed out, the major obstacles to getting to ninety, so it is necessary to have some understanding of their cause and how they may be prevented.

Heart Disease and Strokes

The most vulnerable tissues to wear and tear are the walls of the arteries and veins which over many years are exposed to the stress caused by the pressure of blood being pumped around the circulation for seventy years or more. The damage to the lining of the arteries is known as 'atherosclerosis', where the arteries become narrowed by a porridgey-like substance known as atheroma that contains the fat cholesterol.

There are two important consequences when the arteries to the heart and brain are involved. Firstly, insufficient amounts of blood may reach the tissues, thus depriving them of oxygen which is necessary for their effective functioning. The effect on the heart is to cause a pain in the chest known as angina and in the brain a loss of memory and concentration.

Secondly, and more seriously, a clot or thrombus of sticky

platelets (tiny blood cells) may develop in the already narrowed artery so the blood flow to the relevant organ (or part of it) ceases dramatically. If this occurs in the arteries to the heart, the result is a heart attack (or coronary thrombosis) and in the arteries to the brain, a major stroke.

Everyone has some degree of atherosclerosis: in the western world it can be viewed as almost normal, no different from a balding head or wrinkled face. Its severity is, however, accelerated in the indolent, the cigarette smoker and those with raised blood pressure. These exacerbating factors are, however, modifiable, while the free flow of blood can be promoted by taking aspirin to reduce the stickiness of the blood and, where appropriate, cholesterol-lowering drugs to reduce the amount of atheroma. Hence heart attacks and strokes may be preventable, or at least postponable.

Cancer

The situation is rather different with the third major obstacle to getting to ninety: cancer. The risk of this also increases with age, probably because the body's immune system loses the ability to identify and destroy malignant cells. Unlike the circulatory disorders, cancer cannot be prevented by modifying one's lifestyle (with the obvious exception of smoking) or taking medication. Rather, the possibilities of prevention lie almost entirely with 'screening', where cases are picked up at an early enough stage for them to be readily curable.

The next three chapters examine the many ways life can be prolonged by preventing the Big Three diseases. The effort involved in 'living longer' may appear complex and time consuming. It is not. Most, as will become clear, is little more than commonsense.

PART 1

LIVING LONGER

It would be truly wonderful if there were a rejuvenation pill that would keep our bones strong, our blood flowing and the brain ticking over. But there is not, so we must resort to more devious means to maximise our chances of making it to ninety. The principles, however, are easy enough to grasp and for the most part turn out to be little more than common sense.

We start with what we can do for ourselves and in A Sober Life we examine the degree to which regular exercise, abstaining from tobacco and alcohol and eating sensibly may, or may not, protect us from the sniper fire of heart disease, strokes and cancer. Screening, the second of our approaches, examines how, by catching serious diseases like raised blood pressure and cancer early enough for them to be cured, we can add a decade or more to our lives. And lastly, drugs being potent chemicals can keep the blood flowing through the arteries and the hormone levels high. They may not be the elixir of life, but used judiciously can, like screening, usefully extend the lifespan.

1

A SOBER LIFE

Sobriety is widely believed to hold the key to a long and healthy life. There is, however, no point in giving up life's pleasures to no purpose, so it is interesting to note that whereas two aspects of a sober life – regular exercise and abstaining from tobacco – are indeed useful, a further two – teetotalism and a 'healthy' diet – are much less so.

Exercise

Exercise is bunk. If you are healthy, you don't need it: if you are sick you shouldn't take it.

Henry Ford, 1863–1947

Henry Ford may have lived to the ripe age of eighty-four by following this maxim, but he was lucky. There can be no doubt that those who take regular exercise live longer than those who do not. This may be obvious, but the most interesting finding of recent years is that it applies not just to the fanatical but also to those who take moderate daily exercise. This might seem difficult to prove, but when the fitness of 10,000 middle-aged men and women was assessed by determining how long they could walk against a treadmill before dropping out from exhaustion, it was found that over the succeeding ten years the very fit did best but only a small margin separated them from the moderately fit. The least fit did terribly, with a threefold increased risk of dying before their time. The effect of exercise is to increase the adaptability of the heart and lungs, thus compensating for the decline in function that occurs with age as well as opening up 'spare' arteries to the heart muscle, ensuring that blood will reach the tissues. Hence exercise both reduces the likelihood of a heart attack and, by lowering the blood pressure, reduces the risk of stroke.

The elastic limits of physical fitness are enormous. The geriatric marathon record is held by a seventy-nine-year-old man who completed the gruelling course in just under four hours. This is, to be sure, twice as long as it takes a superbly fit young man (or woman), but compared to the unfit of any age is still remarkable. It is also unachievable for all except the most fanatical of exercise enthusiasts, so it is more interesting to focus on realistic goals. Moderate fitness is our aim.

The best way to approach the exercise question is to take someone who has been inactive for a decade or so and consider how to improve his physical condition. The first priority is to increase the flexibility and strength of the muscles. Here standard exercise routines learnt at a keep fit class or taken from a book or video supplemented by working out in the gym are all quite straightforward. Muscle strength can be improved at any age, indeed when ten frail eighty-year-olds were put through a course of such exercises subsequent testing revealed their strength had almost doubled.

Once the muscles are more supple and stronger, it is time to move on to aerobic exercise of sufficient intensity to stress the heart. This can usually be achieved by a brisk sixty-minute walk every day. And how brisk is brisk? Probably between four and six miles an hour, that is walking a mile in around fifteen minutes. The brisk walk is, of course, only a benchmark – one might as easily play tennis or go ballroom dancing every day.

Alternatively, more vigorous exercise can be taken for a shorter period, such as jogging for twenty minutes every other day, preceded and followed by fifteen-minute periods for warming up and slowing down. The necessary level of exercise to achieve fitness is that which pushes the heart rate up to 120 beats a minutes, which is easily calculated holding a watch in one hand and placing the other over the heart pounding in the chest.

But this type of rigorous exercise certainly has its dangers. First, more than half of the participants in over-enthusiastic jogging programmes may be incapacitated by strained ligaments and stress fractures. Next, and more seriously, there is always the possibility that stressing the heart can induce either a heart attack or some serious disturbance of heart rhythm. It is estimated that this type of vigorous exercise probably increases the risk of a cardiac episode (i.e. some heart problem) by a factor of four while the person is exercising. Rather ominously, it has been suggested that exercise at this level should be considered as 'the basis of a happier life rather than a means to a longer one'. It is possible to take a more positive view by first getting a check-up, which might at least show if there is evidence of heart disease. After that it is a matter of taking one's chances. In the United States, older joggers are often advised not to go out alone but take a partner – so if misfortune does strike there is someone on hand to raise the alarm and, if appropriate, start resuscitation. Not that jogging does not have other dangers. In recent years there have been reports of 'jogger's nipple' – an irritation of the nipples caused by friction against a sweat-drenched shirt. Then there have been cases of 'jogger's testicles' – a sensation of discomfort attributed to gravitational pull in those with inadequate support. And worst of all, 'jogger's penile frostbite' in those whose dedication takes them out in sub-zero temperatures.

The important lesson about exercise that cannot be emphasised too strongly is that only a narrow margin of benefit divides the seriously from the moderately fit. In practical terms, the amount of exercise that can prolong life is what most sensible people take anyhow – a brisk walk for an hour or more a day.

Smoking

I smoke continuously, sometimes in the middle of the night. And I drink anything I can lay my hands on.

Joe Smart on his one hundredth birthday

There is no point in rehearsing the potential harm of tobacco. Joe Smart was exceptionally fortunate not to have suffered from lung cancer, bronchitis, emphysema or heart disease in his seventies or even earlier. Those who never started, or stopped after a few years, did themselves a favour.

The question posed by the small band still smoking over the age of sixty is whether it is still worthwhile giving up and, if not, whether switching to a pipe or cigars is a viable alternative. The depressing news for smokers is that it probably is worth quitting at any age, as this slows the steady loss of lung function that afflicts smokers. There are, as always, considerable differences between individuals in their susceptibility to lung damage from tobacco, but on average it seems that the non-smoker at seventy-five will still have three-quarters of his useful lung capacity, the persistent smoker about a quarter. This is a monumental difference. It is less clear whether it is worthwhile switching to another source of nicotine like a pipe or cigar. These are held to be less dangerous than cigarettes, but probably because cigar and pipe smokers 'puff' rather than inhale. A committed cigarette smoker who makes the switch is likely to carry on inhaling and so continues to damage his airways.

The prospects of quitting, at least relatively painlessly, have been transformed in recent years by the proliferation of alternative ways of getting nicotine into the bloodstream – as a nasal spray, chewing gum or, most popular of all, patches. That said, there can be no argument against the occasional cigar and there is some consolation in the recent observation that nicotine, by stimulating the neuro-transmitters in the brain, can remarkably improve intellectual performance.

A 'Healthy' Diet

Whereas the benefits of moderate exercise and stopping smoking are readily demonstrable, those of a 'healthy' diet are only of marginal importance. This may sound surprising and requires some explanation. The prevailing nutritional wisdom runs along the following lines: saturated fat in meat, milk and dairy foods pushes up the level of cholesterol in the blood, thus exacerbating the atheroma that narrows the arteries; salt 'overloads' the circulation and so raises the blood pressure, and too much sugar leads to overweight and diabetes. Contrariwise, bread, potatoes and vegetables keep the bowels moving regularly and, so it is claimed, prevent cancer, varicose veins, piles and much else. Ergo, 'a healthy diet' requires eating less fat, salt and sugar and consuming lots of fruit, vegetables and high fibre foods instead.

This all sounds plausible enough and certainly the imagery of, for example, fatty foods like bacon and eggs furring up the arteries is powerful enough. There are several reasons, however, why one should be sceptical. First, people do not eat 'diets', they eat food and derive a lot of pleasure from it. Fat adds subtlety to the taste of many foods which is why it is so popular and why, one suspects, puritanical health enthusiasts feel we should eat less of it. Next, we live in a society where for the first time most people live out their natural lifespan, so what we eat cannot be that harmful. Indeed, the two countries with the longest lifespan, Sweden and Japan, could not have more dissimilar patterns of food consumption, so again, diet alone is unlikely to be an important determinant of health. Then, it is actually very difficult to lower the blood pressure or cholesterol levels by changing one's diet because so many other mechanisms are involved in ensuring these remain within very narrow limits. We certainly could not survive if the blood pressure fluctuated markedly depending on how much salt we consume from one day to the next. It is only by going to extremes – by massively over-consuming salt or eating hardly any at all – that the blood pressure can be altered.

Nonetheless, the medical belief in the virtues of a 'healthy' diet is for the moment virtually unshakeable and it is currently very common for people to be told that they should for their own good stop eating this and start eating that. Such medical intrusion in the simple pleasures of the table is quite unwarranted and those who, quite rightly, resent such gratuitous advice will be interested in the following:

(i) *The link between fat and heart disease* was investigated in the largest experiment ever conducted in the history of medicine. At a cost of £100 million, 12,000 men were divided into two groups to see whether cutting down on meat, milk and dairy foods might prevent their risk of a heart attack. After ten years, the rate of heart disease in those who had been forced to make these radical changes to their diet was precisely the same as in those who had not. Nonetheless, fish and particularly oily fish such as mackerel certainly reduce the stickiness of the blood and it is possible that if consumed regularly, say twice a week, this may reduce the risk of a clot forming in the arteries and thus prevent a heart attack.

(ii) *Salt and raised blood pressure* The main effect of not adding salt to cooking is to reduce the amount that is subsequently excreted in the urine – and so has no effect on the total amount in the body. Besides making food unpalatable for most, even extreme salt reduction has no sustainable influence on the blood pressure and indeed in some people can produce a paradoxical increase.

(iii) *Sugar, overweight and diabetes* The link between sugar and overweight is commonly made, with the implication that it must be entirely transformed into fat. This is not true. Sugar is only implicated in obesity because it makes food more attractive and so people eat more than they should. Sugar does not cause diabetes, which is due to relative or absolute deficiency of the hormone insulin.

(iv) *Fibre and the bowel* This is one of the few instances where changing one's dietary habits does have a clear and recognisable effect on how the body works. Fibre,

11

whether in the form of high fibre foods such as brown bread, potatoes and bran or as a fibre supplement, increases the frequency and loosens the consistency of the stool and is thus an effective treatment for constipation and may be helpful for those who suffer from an irritable bowel.

The putative benefits of 'healthy' eating are much less than promised. The message is well rehearsed if unexciting: 'Moderation in all things'. Make a virtue out of variety, worry more about whether your food is fresh and well cooked than what it is doing to you and little harm can result. It is safe to say that reading cook books is much more worthwhile than following nutritional advice of any sort.

'Sensible' Drinking

Having won the campaign against tobacco, health enthusiasts have subsequently switched their attention to the alleged dangers of alcohol. Erudite committees, ignorant of Louis Pasteur's famous dictum 'wine is the most helpful and hygienic of beverages', have drawn up guidelines of what constitutes 'sensible' drinking. Their proposed limits should be treated with considerable scepticism.

Certainly, heavy drinking, that is half a bottle of whisky or more a day, is very destructive but those with this level of drinking do not need advice, but professional help. At the other extreme, teetotalism also has its drawbacks, as alcohol has a protective effect on the heart. Hence those who enjoy wine with their dinner in the evening will fare at least as well, if not better, than those with mineral water on the table.

This has not stopped experts laying down the law as to what they consider to be the upper limit of safe drinking – 21 units of alcohol a week for men and 15 a week for women. It is difficult to remember how much alcohol there is in a 'unit', but as a general guide it means a glass of wine or half a pint of beer, so if these recommendations are adhered to, we should limit ourselves to a couple of glasses of wine (or its equivalent) a day. This seems a bit mean, as indeed it is, and is a long way off what is needed to get slightly merry. It must be stressed that there is no serious scientific basis for these recommendations, which over the years have always been revised downwards. There seems little doubt that people can double this intake with no obvious untoward effect.

Conclusion

It turns out that it is not necessary to lead *that* sober a life to keep fit and raise the odds for a longer life. It can be reduced to three positive and three negative messages.

Positively:
- Spend an hour in the gym twice a week and take a brisk walk (or its equivalent) every day
- Enjoy at least a couple of glasses of wine every evening
- Try and eat fish at least twice a week.

Negatively:
- Over-vigorous exercise is to be discouraged because of the risk it poses to the joints and heart
- Don't bother fiddling around with what you eat
- Stop smoking.

Of course, there is always the feeling that perhaps one should be doing more, but it must be stressed these axioms are the only ones substantiated by convincing scientific evidence.

2

SCREENING

'Screening' is the second method of increasing the chances of Living Longer. Its purpose is self-evident: to identify a serious illness before it becomes apparent, in the hope of catching it early enough for it to be more readily treatable. Screening is the medical term for 'searching'. The doctor is searching for disease in the apparently healthy. In most he will find nothing, or nothing of much consequence. In a few, however, the blood pressure or cholesterol level will be found to be too high which, if treated, might avert a heart attack or stroke in the future, or special tests may detect cancer at an early enough stage for it to be curable. The putative benefits of screening are plausible enough, but one must be aware of its limitations. It can only find what the scrutiny of the doctor and the sensitivity of the test can reveal and so is limited to detecting those diseases that can be found quite easily. Put another way, there are many illnesses for which there is no effective screening test and so, by definition, they cannot be detected early.

Then there are the limits of the tests themselves which can have 'false positive' or 'false negative' results. A false positive is where a condition is identified which is not in fact present; for example, a suspicious shadow on a chest X-ray may turn out after much further investigation to be unimportant. A false negative is where a chest X-ray appears normal, but fails to detect a small tumour which then goes undiagnosed. Here the person being screened may be reassured there is nothing wrong when in fact there is.

I mention these limitations not to discourage screening but to warn that it can generate needless anxiety, while the reassurance of a clean bill of health can be misleading. While the benefits of screening for an individual can be indisputable, the likelihood of being the person to benefit is very small, while the possibility of being needlessly worried is quite high.

In Britain, two grades of screening are available – a basic one provided by the National Health Service and a deluxe 'private' version which involves a physical check-up, lots of blood tests and investigations. There is a lot of enthusiasm for screening in private medicine as it provides the opportunity to run a series of investigations, which most of the time will be completely normal. This is a lucrative business. Those not willing or able to 'go private' should not be perturbed for, as will be seen, it offers little more than that which is available on the Health Service.

Health Service Screening

The Blood Pressure

As everyone knows, raised blood pressure (or hypertension) is a major risk factor for strokes, a devastating catastrophe which can be avoided by dropping into the doctor's surgery once every two years and having one's blood pressure measured. The question as to how 'high' the blood pressure has to be to merit treatment is discussed in the next chapter.

Cholesterol Levels

There is currently great enthusiasm for measuring the cholesterol levels in the blood, actively encouraged by the pharmaceutical industry, who hope that doctors will then prescribe one or other of their expensive cholesterol-lowering drugs. The benefits of cholesterol lowering are much less clear-cut than for treating raised blood pressure, but there is no doubt that appropriate medication is indicated in those whose levels are markedly elevated. This is discussed in the next chapter.

The purpose of screening to detect raised blood pressure and cholesterol is to protect people against the sniper fire from the two major circulatory disorders – stroke and heart disease respectively. Protection against the third sniper – cancer – requires specialised tests to identify tumours of the cervix, breast and prostate early enough for them to be readily treatable.

Cancer screening

Cervical cancer: The shape and appearance of cells removed from the cervix with a smear test can identify those that might turn malignant. The problem, as always, is that not all the 'abnormalities' so detected will go on to cause mischief in the future. So some women with abnormal smears will be treated for a problem that, if left alone, may never have materialised. Women should probably have a cervical smear once every three to five years.

Breast cancer: The most reliable method of detecting this much-feared cancer early is with an X-ray of the breast known as a mammogram – otherwise known as a 'boob squash', because the breast has to be compressed between two metal plates to get a good 'picture'.

The mammogram, like cervical smears, can be ambiguous, making it difficult to decide what is a potential cancer and what is not, so about one in a hundred women in whom an abnormality is detected have to have it biopsied. Even then, it can be difficult to be absolutely certain as to whether the lump is cancerous, so erring on the side of caution some women will be treated for a 'cancer' they don't have. The compensation is that breast cancer correctly diagnosed and treated at its earliest stages is usually considered to be cured.

Prostate cancer: Tumours of the prostate gland at the base of the bladder have the unfortunate tendency not to cause symptoms until the cancer is quite advanced, so in over a third of cases it is already widespread at the time of diagnosis – which is obviously bad news.

The ability to detect prostate cancer early has much improved since the discovery that a blood test for a chemical secreted by the gland (the prostate specific antigen, or PSA) is elevated in those in whom the cancer is still confined to the gland when it is still potentially curable. If the PSA is raised, the diagnosis can then be confirmed with a scan and a biopsy. Treatment requires either a major operation (radical prostatectomy) to remove the gland in its entirety, or radiotherapy (X-ray treatment).

As with all forms of cancer screening, the benefits are not quite as straightforward as might appear. The problem is that over the age of seventy, most men will have some malignant cells in their prostate but in the vast majority they will either not progress to threaten their lives or they may succumb to some other illness, in which case the presence of the cancer cells in the gland is irrelevant. There is thus inevitably the danger that having one's PSA measured may result in unnecessary treatment.

In summary then, five serious conditions can, in theory at least, be avoided by one or other of the screening tests available on the NHS:

- Stroke – blood pressure
- Heart disease – cholesterol
- Cancer of the cervix – cervical smear
- Cancer of the breast – mammogram
- Cancer of the prostate – PSA.

If the range of diseases detectable by screening is to be increased, it is necessary to opt for the deluxe 'private' version – for which obviously one has to pay good money.

Private Screening

Private screening is a lucrative business, exploiting many people's quite natural apprehension about their health. Considerable effort is therefore made to convey the impression of giving value for money. An attentive and well-dressed doctor goes through the ritual of performing a thorough physical examination doing lots of blood tests and other investigations, but importantly there are only a few instances where this is of any value over and above the screening tests available on the health service. These are outlined below.

Abdominal aortic aneurysm (AAA)

The abdominal aorta which runs along the back of the abdomen against the spine is the major artery carrying blood to the kidneys, liver and down into the legs. When its wall becomes weak it billows out to form an aneurysm, which may burst with predictably catastrophic consequences – the blood pressure falls, blood leaks into surrounding tissues, there is severe abdominal pain and collapse. If the patient can be got to hospital in time an operation (in which the diseased aneurysm is cut out and replaced with an artificial artery or 'graft') may be possible. It is, however, a tricky business and not all patients make it. It would seem more sensible to have the operation before this happens, which means, of course, detecting the aneurysm before it bursts.

It is possible to self-diagnose an aortic aneurysm by placing the hand flat on the tummy while in bed at night. If the pulsation is particularly strong and appears to move outwards then a visit to the family doctor is called for which will confirm or exclude the diagnosis. The only other method of early diagnosis is during the systematic physical examination which is part of private screening. Those in whom the aneurysm is found to be greater than 5 cm in diameter usually have it repaired while smaller ones may be observed to see if they get any larger.

Chest X-ray for smokers

The doctor conducting the private screening will, following the physical examination, order a large number of blood tests, as well as measuring the lung function and assessing the heart with an ECG and chest X-ray. The chances that these investigations will identify some illness that was not previously known about and requires treatment are virtually zero and there is no need to fear that by not having them, some serious disease will go undetected. The one exception is a chest X-ray in smokers. Chest X-rays are easy to do and lung cancer is common, so it would seem advisable for smokers (and indeed ex-smokers) to have a yearly chest X-ray in the hope that the cancer will be detected early enough for it to be cured. Initially it was thought that most of the cancers detected in this way would be too far advanced for anything to be done about them. More recently, however, it has become clear that regular X-rays can after all be of value, with three-quarters of those in whom the cancer is diagnosed in its earlier stages surviving for five years or more.

Those who opt for private screening can also be tested for two further cancers.

Cancer of the ovary

Ovarian cancer can spread within the pelvis long before any symptoms become apparent, so by the time the diagnosis is made it is often 'too late'. It can, however, be detected early with an ultrasound scan which outlines the structure of the ovaries. The number of positive findings is low. In a study of 800 women, fifty were thought to have some abnormality; thirty-nine of these underwent surgery (which is required to find out exactly what it going on), revealing only one cancer.

Cancer of the large bowel

There are two ways in which this serious cancer can be detected. Firstly, the lining of the lower bowel can be inspected with a sigmoidoscope in the hope of either finding a cancer in the earliest stages or a benign tumour or polyp, which if left alone might subsequently turn malignant. Secondly, bowel cancer often leaks blood into the gut – too little to be seen by ordinary inspection but detectable by placing a specimen of stool on a specially prepared piece of paper called haemoccult. Those with a positive result are then further investigated, either with a special X-ray of the large bowel or a colonoscopy (the passing of a fibreoptic tube up through the rectum and round the bowel through which the surgeon can see the source of bleeding). Again, the number of positive findings is very low. Eighteen thousand people whose stools were tested in this way produced seventy-seven 'positive results', twelve of whom had cancer – nine at a curative stage – and one was missed.

Is It Worth It?

Screening can turn sensible people into hypochondriacs. The whole process of attending for tests is in itself quite worrying. When these turn up ambiguous results requiring further investigation, it is easy to see how a lot of anxiety can be generated especially as these investigations – such as biopsies and special X-rays – are in themselves quite traumatic. Finally, there is the problem of over-treatment, as there is the obvious tendency to think that all 'abnormalities' must be treated if screening is to be justified. Consequently, many of those with 'raised' blood pressure or cholesterol levels take medication for years to no purpose, while running the risk of experiencing their side-effects. Others may be told they have 'cancer' (with all that implies) and submit to radical treatment for a disease which if left undiscovered would not have altered their life expectancy. The only advice that can be given in these circumstances is that if an abnormality is found, the question should be asked "what will happen if we do nothing about it?" And if one is not entirely satisfied with the result, there is always the option of seeking a second opinion.

Having said all this, there can be no doubt that screening certainly does benefit some individuals. Despite the low rate of disease revealed by screening, nonetheless the seven out of 18,000 individuals who did turn out to have curable bowel cancer in the study cited above, probably owe their lives to it.

Screening can be useful – but who should have what test and how often? Clearly some sort of discrimination is required, as it would be quite possible to spend a lot of time being screened for one disease or other, which is not a recipe for a happy life.

Who?

Theoretically, anyone might benefit from screening tests, but those in whom a family member has had one or other of the diseases being screened for – especially if it developed when they were still relatively young (less than sixty) – are particularly likely to do so. Both the raised cholesterol levels that may contribute to heart disease and the various forms of cancer detectable by screening are in part genetically determined, so if one or other occurs in a close relative, this suggests you may be at greater risk which should strengthen your resolve to have the screening test done.

What For?

This will obviously depend on your sex and, again, if there is a strong family history of heart disease or cancer.

How Often?

Though the range of tests might seem daunting, a suggested screening programme is fairly straightforward:

- Once only (NHS) – cholesterol
- Annually (privately) – chest X-ray for smokers and ex-smokers
- Two years (NHS) – blood pressure
- Three years (NHS) – mammogram, cervical smear and PSA
- Five years (private) – physical examination (to detect an aortic aneurysm), ovarian ultrasound, sigmoid oscopy and stool blood testing.

Thus, if you are a male you should probably drop in to visit the family doctor to have your cholesterol measured on one occasion and once every three years to have your blood pressure tested and a PSA test. If you are a woman you too should have your blood pressure measured regularly. You will have been invited to have a cervical smear and mammogram on a regular basis up to the age of sixty-five and it may be worthwhile to have a couple more – which can be requested – after that. So, it's not that complicated. The question as to whether you should in addition have a private screening, perhaps every five years, will, of course, depend on your circumstances.

Where?

Most of the screening tests, as pointed out, are readily available on the health service. There are, however, some important points that need to be made. The easy tests, like blood pressure and cholesterol, can be done quite simply. There is a national screening programme for cervical and breast cancer, where women are invited every five years to attend for a test. The rest are certainly available, but not routinely, so have to be requested, as in "my brother has just been diagnosed as having prostate cancer, should I have a PSA test?" Further, if there is a strong family history of ovarian or bowel cancer and this is shown to have a genetic component, then it is usually possible also to have the relevant test on the Health Service. This would essentially restrict the advantages of private screening to regular chest X-rays for smokers and the physical examination to look for an abnormal aortic aneurysm. The main advantage of private screening, however, is undoubtedly its convenience and thoroughness, so people can have all the relevant tests at one go and then at appropriate intervals thereafter.

Ultimately the question of deciding which level of screening is appropriate will vary from one person to another – how important is it for him or her to know that they have done as much as they can to pick up potentially lethal but curable diseases, or how necessary the reassurance that all seems to be well.

3

DRUGS THAT PREVENT DISEASE

The flow of blood to the brain and heart is impeded in two of the Big Three illnesses – stroke and heart disease. Clearly every effort should be made to prevent this, which may require taking some potent drug to lower the blood pressure, reduce the cholesterol level (and thus the narrowing of the arteries) or reduce the stickiness of the blood with a daily dose of aspirin. In women, Hormone Replacement Therapy has a similar effect, as well as preventing the thinning of the bones known as osteoporosis.

The best established of these 'drugs that prevent disease' are those for the treatment of raised blood pressure (hypertension), with which we start.

Hypertension

Raised blood pressure can be bad news. It can burst an artery in the brain, rendering its victim paralysed or speechless, or cause heart failure by requiring the heart to contract too vigorously when pushing the blood round the circulation.

What is 'Blood Pressure'?

When the heart contracts, the valves open and the forceful thrust of blood out into the major arteries is known as the *systolic* pressure. When the blood hits the walls of the arteries they expand slightly and then, like a rubber band, ping back into shape propelling the blood onwards – this is the *diastolic* pressure. The blood pressure is thus recorded as the *systolic* pressure (which has an upper limit of about 140 mm of mercury) over the *diastolic* (90 mm of mercury) – which is written as 140/90.

There is, however, no clear cut-off point that distinguishes the 'normal' from the 'raised' – though as a rule of thumb, a diastolic pressure between 100 and 110 is 'mild' hypertension, between 110 and 120 is 'moderate' and anything over 120 is 'severe'.

Hypertension may cause headaches and ringing in the ears, but mostly it is symptomless and so can only be diagnosed by visiting the family doctor to have the blood pressure checked – which should preferably be done every two years. It varies naturally during the day, so do not be alarmed if a single recording is 'too high'. The blood pressure has to be raised consistently on three separate occasions, preferably a month apart, before treatment can be justified. The anxiety of visiting the surgery almost invariably pushes the blood pressure upwards so it is sensible to buy your own machine which will more reliably and accurately reflect the response to treatment.

Treatment

The several ways of lowering the blood pressure without having to take medication have already been discussed in A Sober Life. Contrary to common advice, there is no justification in cutting down on salt intake, as it is ineffective and renders food unpalatable. Raised blood pressure in the overweight, however, will often return to normal by the simple expedient of losing a few stones. Regular exercise is highly recommended, as it increases the number and diameter of the arteries in the muscle, thus reducing the pressure with which the blood has to be pumped around the circulation.

The simplest form of drug treatment is the mild water tablet or diuretic known as bendrofluazide, which is usually well tolerated but can 'bring out' diabetes and cause erectile impotence in men. If this is insufficient, then further drugs will be necessary, including betablockers (such as atenolol) or calcium antagonists (such as verapamil) or ACE inhibitors. Once the decision has been made to treat raised blood pressure, then treatment should theoretically continue indefinitely. In some, however, raised blood pressure may return to normal so it is worthwhile, especially in those with milder levels, to stop treatment after a couple of years for a month or so to see what happens.

In summary then:

- Have your blood pressure checked every two years
- Do not start treatment unless it has been found to be raised on at least three separate occasions
- Make an effort to monitor your own blood pressure, as otherwise you may end up taking more treatment than is necessary
- After a couple of years, discuss the possibility of stopping treatment to see if the blood pressure stays down.

'High' Cholesterol

The rationale for lowering cholesterol levels runs along similar lines to those for treating blood pressure. Just as hypertension is usually symptomless, so regular blood pressure checks are necessary to find those who need treating, so a raised cholesterol level in the blood can only be detected by doing a blood test. Those in whom it is found to be elevated either need to be on a low-fat diet or to take cholesterol-lowering drugs. The analogy can, however, be misleading as hypertension is a much more powerful risk factor for stroke than cholesterol is for heart disease. Indeed, the identification and treatment of raised cholesterol is only of value in a small minority in whom it is markedly elevated (above 10) – though regrettably there is considerable pressure on doctors to treat levels lower than this. Next, the cholesterol, like the blood pressure, tends to increase with age, so what might be deemed 'high' in the young can be quite normal in a sixty-year-old. Further, it is not at all easy to lower the cholesterol with a low-fat diet, which anyhow requires giving up many pleasurable foods. Drugs are certainly much more effective, but can have serious side-effects including causing depression.

In summary, the benefits of lowering the cholesterol and preventing a heart attack are considerably less than lowering the blood pressure and preventing stroke. Those in whom a close relative has had a heart attack should certainly have their cholesterol measured, but for everyone else the best advice is probably to forget about it: do not bother to have your cholesterol measured, and if it is found to be 'elevated' resist any moves to have it treated with drugs.

Aspirin

Aspirin is the 'wonder drug of the century'. Its pain relieving and anti-inflammatory properties have been known for over a century, but in addition it was discovered in the mid-seventies to prevent the formation of blood clots in the arteries by reducing the stickiness of the platelet cells. Thus an aspirin a day should improve the blood flow and reduce the risk of both heart attacks and stroke.

There is no doubt that when taken by those who already have had a heart attack or stroke, aspirin markedly reduces the risk of having another. It would thus seem eminently sensible that, as it is both cheap and relatively innocuous (though it can irritate the stomach), to advise everyone to take a small dose every day to prevent one or other of these medical catastrophes in the first place. The question is whether it works and here there is a difference of opinion. In the United States, a study of 3,000 physicians found that those given an aspirin daily did much better than those given a placebo, with a lower risk of both heart disease and stroke. But the results of a similar study in Britain, this time involving 500 doctors, failed to show any benefit. So what to do? A possible compromise might be that those at 'high risk' who have a strong family history of circulatory disorders should take a regular daily dose of aspirin as a preventive measure. However, heart attacks and strokes are best avoided and the risks of aspirin are probably acceptable, so it is difficult to quarrel with those who, with a careful attitude to their future health, feel they should take aspirin regularly.

Hormone Replacement Therapy

Hormone Replacement Therapy (HRT) is the most natural and physiological of the 'drugs that prevent disease', as it involves literally 'replacing' the female hormones oestrogen and progesterone, whose levels decline precipitously following the menopause. Its benefits can be divided into the immediate and the long term.

- *Immediate*: HRT relieves the acute symptoms of the menopause, providing relief from hot flushes, promoting a general sense of well-being, preventing mood swings and maintaining vaginal secretions that make sexual intercourse more pleasurable. If a woman stops taking HRT after several years, the symptoms will to a greater or lesser extent return – which is a good enough reason to continue to take it indefinitely.
- *Long term*: Long-term benefits of HRT include the prevention of heart attacks, strokes and osteoporosis. Women are less prone to heart disease than men because oestrogen has a protective effect on the lining of the arteries. This is likely to be extended by taking HRT after the menopause and indeed it reduces heart disease by almost a half, with a similar reduction in the number of strokes. HRT also seems to have a more generalised effect, halving the rate of untimely death in those taking it, compared to those who do not. This is all impressive, but probably overestimates the benefits as its use is most widespread amongst the higher social classes who tend to do better in health terms generally.

The other long-term benefit of HRT is the prevention of osteoporosis. Following the menopause, the bones become thinner, increasing the likelihood of sustaining a fracture of the wrist or hips or collapse of the vertebrae. These are serious complications and may require a major operation such as a total hip replacement. So even a modest reduction in the risk of fracture is to be welcomed. HRT is the only certain way of keeping the bones as strong as possible, but this may require taking it well into one's seventies and eighties, when the incidence of fractures due to osteoporosis starts to rise significantly.

So what's the catch? There are two. The menopause frees women of the tedium of the monthly period, for which in the past many were very grateful. Regrettably, and for obvious reasons, those taking HRT will continue having periods though it is important to know that there are some types in which this does not happen. More seriously, HRT marginally increases the risk of breast cancer. Breast cancer is a hormone-dependent tumour and women are at greatest risk whose breasts are exposed to oestrogen for a long time, i.e. those who have an early puberty and a late menopause. If one 'defers' the menopause with hormone replacement, then the likelihood is that the risk of breast cancer will increase still further.

So what to conclude? Women who take HRT gain substantial tangible benefits in terms of the immediate reduction of the distressing symptoms of the menopause, which may well outweigh the increased risk of a potentially serious disease later on. Beyond this the dilemma is whether it is worthwhile to take hormones regularly to prevent something such as a heart attack or a fracture due to osteoporosis that may never happen, while at the same time increasing the risk of breast cancer, which also might never happen.

Living Longer: Conclusions

The only certain way of prolonging life is to prevent or defer the three Big Illnesses – heart disease, strokes and cancer. These are all in their different ways age-determined disorders – that is, the older one gets, the higher the risk. There is nothing that one can do to stop getting older and thus the best one can do to prevent these disorders or catch them early is to combine one or other of the approaches outlined in A Sober Life, Screening and Drugs That Prevent Disease. These are now summarised below.

Heart Disease

A Sober Life

1. *Exercise*: promotes fitness and slows the decline of heart function by strengthening the heart muscle and 'opening up' the blood vessels.
2. *Diet*: The usual advice to reduce the amount of fat in the diet has little effect on the cholesterol level and thus the accumulation of atheroma in the arteries. However, eating fish regularly may antagonise the clotting ten-

dency of the blood. Alcohol appears to be similarly protective.

3. *Smoking*: Stopping smoking may modestly influence the development of atheroma, but is much more important in keeping the lungs healthy and so increasing the amount of oxygen that can be pushed around the body.

Screening

Both raised blood pressure and a markedly raised cholesterol are risk factors for heart disease and can be readily detected by paying a visit to the family doctor.

Preventive Drugs

The treatment of raised blood pressure and markedly raised cholesterol levels can slow the development of heart disease. Aspirin can certainly prevent heart disease in those who have already experienced one or other of these illnesses, but its preventive effect in those who are otherwise healthy is disputed. Hormone Replacement Therapy also has a protective effect.

Strokes

A Sober Life

1. *Exercise*: reduces the blood pressure which is a major cause of strokes.
2. *Diet*: Reducing the amount of salt in the diet has no

sustainable effect on raised blood pressure. Those who are obese, however, will benefit by losing weight.

3. *Smoking*: Stopping smoking will reduce the risk of a stroke by itself and by encouraging more exercise.

Screening

Screening is much the most effective way of preventing a stroke, by having the blood pressure checked regularly.

Preventive Drugs

Drugs that reduce the blood pressure will prevent a stroke. HRT probably also has a protective role, as does aspirin.

Cancer

A Sober Life

1. *Diet*: There is no evidence that a 'healthy' diet will reduce the risk of cancer.

2. *Smoking*: Stopping smoking markedly reduces the risk of lung cancer, which after ten years is only slightly greater in those who have never smoked.

Screening

Screening provides the best hope of early treatment and cure.

- Lung cancer: an annual chest X-ray
- Breast cancer: a mammogram every three to five years

- Cervical cancer: a cervical smear every three to five years
- Prostate cancer: measurement of the PSA every three to five years
- Colon cancer: sigmoidoscopy and regular testing for blood in the stools
- Ovarian cancer: detectable by ultrasound.

Living Longer turns out to be little more than common sense. Sensible people take regular exercise, but do not overdo it. They enjoy food and drink, but are fairly sceptical about the radical dietary changes encouraged by healthy eating enthusiasts. They have long since given up smoking. They drop in every so often to see the doctor to have their blood pressure checked and if it is raised take their medication religiously. Women are aware of the benefits of taking HRT and submit themselves to a cervical smear and mammogram on a regular basis. Similarly, men are well advised to have a PSA test. Those who wish to do a bit better than this will take an aspirin a day and have a regular 'private' health check-up every five years. And that's it.

PART 2

WHEN THINGS GO WRONG

The goal of Living Longer is highly desirable on many counts, but it is an inescapable fact that for virtually everyone things will go wrong at some time or other. Hence, regrettably, the longer people live, the greater their dependence on modern medicine to keep them healthy and active. This dependence has its problems which can best be minimised by knowing at least a bit about how medicine works – which this section seeks to clarify. Nobody wants to bother their doctor unnecessarily, so it is helpful to have some insight into how to distinguish the 'serious' symptoms that merit medical attention from the trivial. Next, it is also helpful to have some grasp of how doctors decide what is wrong and particularly the reason for all those tests they are so keen on. And finally, it is helpful to have some sense of the various options involved in putting things right. We start with Is it Serious?

4

IS IT SERIOUS?

The sensible thing to do when things go wrong is to make an appointment to see the doctor, though many people do not, hoping their symptoms will just go away. This stoicism is commendable and, of course, many illnesses do just get better. It seems useful nonetheless to try to distinguish minor illnesses and the aches and discomfort of the passing years from those that are potentially more important.

Besides the coughs and sore throats that are easy enough to recognise, there are three major ways in which things can go wrong which will be illustrated with some appropriate case histories.

Is It Serious?

The three criteria

Novelty – Is the symptom new?
Persistence – Have the symptoms lasted for more than two weeks?
Deterioration – Is the symptom getting worse?

---

1. The Acute–Serious

First, there are the acute-serious illnesses – nasty infections, abdominal emergencies such as a perforated bowel, heart attacks, strokes and many more.

- Mr Julian Richards is a sixty-eight-year-old retired building surveyor. He has been rudely healthy all his life until the last few weeks when he has been bothered by an ache in the chest which he attributes to too much spade work on his allotment. He wakes in the middle of the night with a crushing chest pain, feeling very sweaty and gasping for breath.
- Mr Alan Hopkins develops acute vomiting and diarrhoea following the expensive reception for his son's wedding. He is not the only one.

Both Julian Richards (with his heart attack) and Alan Hopkins (with his food poisoning) found their symptoms came on rapidly and acutely and had no doubt of the need to seek prompt medical attention. The same applies to an attack of bronchitis, a flare-up of sciatica, or any serious, 'panic-worthy' symptom – coughing or vomiting blood, fierce pain in the chest or abdomen, acute shortness of breath, loss of consciousness, paralysis or sudden loss of sight. Each of these can have a variety of causes, some more serious than others, but they all deliver the same simple message – the need for an urgent appointment with the doctor or a call to the ambulance service.

2. Chronic–Degenerative

Next come the chronic-degenerative diseases, a harsh term to describe the 'wear and tear' changes in the body: deterioration of vision or hearing, loss of mobility, difficulty in passing urine and so on.

The essence of these persistent or nagging conditions is that though they are a nuisance, people feel essentially 'well in themselves'.

- Mrs Annie Brooks is seventy-two. A founder member of the League of Health and Beauty, she remains an enthusiastic ballroom dancer. She feels fine, but over the last six months has noticed a pain in her left knee after a particularly vigorous session on the dance floor.

Mrs Brooks's pain is almost certainly due to arthritis of the knee, which needs to be sorted out, but there is no doubt about the diagnosis or treatment.

3. Minor, but Equivocal

The acute-serious and chronic-degenerative can be seen as two ends of a spectrum, but most symptoms fall into a third category – 'minor, but equivocal'. Most of the time these represent trivial illnesses, but occasionally they can be more significant.

- Mr Andrew Wilson has been bothered in recent months by a pain in the stomach, which also wakes him early in the morning. He thought it might be indigestion brought on by his regular breakfast of bacon and eggs, but changing to croissant and muesli has made little difference.

- Mrs Julie Lock, aged seventy-five, used to be very active on the local council and now spends most of her time doing voluntary work. She feels tired all the time and, looking back, she wonders how she ever found the time or energy to lead such a busy life.

Andrew Wilson's pain after eating might be a touch of gastritis that would improve with antacids, or it could be a peptic ulcer or something more sinister. Mrs Lock's tiredness may be due to depression (her favourite son has just moved to Australia) or it may be the first sign that something is seriously amiss.

These 'equivocal' symptoms cover a wide range:

- common complaints such as headache, cough or constipation
- symptoms that can too readily be put down to 'ageing' – aches and pains, breathlessness, or loss of energy
- something 'worrying', like a pain in the chest or abdomen.

It is obviously necessary to know how to distinguish between the 'trivial' and the 'significant' causes of these equivocal symptoms. How can one tell? Irrespective of what the complaint might be, there are three cardinal criteria which strongly suggest that the symptom might be important. They are:

(i) *When the symptom is new*: If the nagging pain in your chest is similar to others you have had over the years, the likelihood is that it is not desperately important. If it is the first time there is a greater likelihood that it is significant.

(ii) *When the symptom persists*: Most illnesses are self-limiting, that is, they get better of their own accord – sometimes before a proper diagnosis has been made. Therefore, giving a new symptom a few days to see whether it just goes away is usually permissible. If it does not, medical attention should be sought.

(iii) *When the symptom is getting worse*: This can apply to symptoms that markedly deteriorate over a day or two, or a longer period such as a week or a month. Again, if this is the case, there should be little delay in obtaining a medical opinion.

Doctors instinctively apply these criteria of novelty, persistence, and deterioration as a sort of red-alert system to distinguish the trivial from the serious, recognising that any equivocal symptoms may herald a potentially important or treatable condition. It is to these that I now turn.

'Common' Complaints

Headache

Headache is one of the commonest pains for which patients seek medical advice. It is usually due to a viral illness (such as influenza) or infection or inflammation of the many structures in the skull, such as the sinuses, teeth and jaw joints, but three commonly recognised types have quite characteristic features:

(i) *Tension headache*: This arises from the back of the neck and spreads up and over the skull. It is often described as a sensation of pressure and is usually caused by tension in the muscles in the back of the neck. This may be due to arthritis in the cervical spine pressing on the nerves, but is commonly a symptom of tension or anxiety.

(ii) *Migraines*: Migraines are confined to one or other side of the head and are often preceded by unusual visual changes. The patient has an aversion to bright lights and seeks comfort in a darkened room.

(iii) *Cluster headaches*: These can last for up to a week at a time, are often located around the orbit of one eye and are strongly associated with stress or overtiredness.

All this is pretty straightforward and, as these types of headaches tend to recur, sufferers usually have no difficulty in recognising them. They also illustrate how any single symptom is highly specific. Thus, saying 'I have a headache' by itself means very little, and only when the details are filled in – the character, duration, precipitating and relieving factors of the headache – is it possible to make a precise diagnosis. This specificity of symptoms in turn allows them to be distinguished from two rarer, and more serious, types:

(iv) *Temporal arteritis*: [An inflammation of the artery (arteritis) on either side of the temple (temporal).] This headache is localised either on the back of the head or on either side of the skull and there is usually a tenderness on touching the affected part, for example when combing the hair or placing the head on the pillow. It responds – usually quite dramatically – to high doses of steroids. Its importance is that if left untreated, the inflammatory process can involve other arteries, notably those to the eye, leading to sudden loss of vision.

(v) *Brain tumour*: The real fear that many people have of headaches is that they might be the first symptom of a brain tumour. They might be, but this is extremely rare not only because, set against the ubiquity of headache as a symptom, brain tumours are uncommon, but also because they are usually heralded by some more obvious symptom such as an epileptic fit or alteration in vision. Nonetheless, if the headache fulfils the three cardinal criteria of novelty, persistence and deterioration over time, it does need medical attention.

Cough

Most people are rightly suspicious of a chronic cough, which in the first half of the century heralded tuberculosis, but now may be the first symptom of other serious conditions.

(i) *Late onset asthma*: Asthma is commonly perceived as being an illness of childhood and adolescence, but may develop for the first time from the sixties onwards, when it is usually accompanied by wheezing and shortness of breath. Treatment with drugs to dilate the airways and steroids can be dramatically effective.

(ii) *Lung tumour*: Smokers who develop a chronic cough are naturally apprehensive that this may be the first sign of a lung tumour. Although it is in the lap of the gods whether it is still treatable by the time the cough starts, they should bite the bullet and have a chest X-ray.

Symptoms often put down to 'Getting On'

We all get used to knowing how our bodies work, and it is easy to presume that some subtle deterioration may merely reflect the passage of time. This is not always the case.

(i) Aches and pains: Aches and stiffness are usually attributed to being no longer young, especially in the less fit and over-weight who take little exercise and have weak or under-used muscles. Before accepting them stoically as a fact of life, several other conditions should be considered, including polymyalgia rheumatica – pain, tenderness and limitation of movement, especially around the shoulders. This improves dramatically with steroid treatment.

(ii) Shortness of breath: It is common enough to get puffed climbing stairs or running for a bus but in general shortness of breath – particularly if there has never been any problem with the heart or lungs in the past – does need to be investigated. The important causes are:

- *Heart failure*: Here the pumping action of the heart necessary to push blood out of the tissues becomes inefficient and fluid collects in the lungs, so the blood receives insufficient oxygen. This may be due to poor contraction of the heart muscle. Water tablets (or diuretics) purge the excess fluid from the lungs.
- *Lung disease*: If the shortness of breath is associated with a wheeze the diagnosis could be 'late onset asthma', which responds well to drugs that dilate the airways.

(iii) Tiredness: The commonest cause of tiredness is psychological. It is natural to feel at times that life is a bit depressing and pointless, which is often experienced as a sense of lassitude. Further, the recovery from any acute illness such as flu or bronchitis can often be associated with a sense of tiredness. There are, however, important remediable physical causes that need to be considered. Many drugs can induce a sense of tiredness and this is particularly true of the betablockers used in the treatment of raised blood pressure. It may also be a symptom of heart failure, an over- or under-active thyroid, or early diabetes or anaemia.

Worrying Pains in the Chest or Abdomen

(i) Chest pains: Many problems of the muscles, lungs or gullet can give rise to a pain in the chest, but the most important are those due to reduced blood flow to the heart muscle. If they are ignored or misunderstood, the patient may not take the necessary steps to prevent a heart attack. The characteristic heart pain – angina – is 'crushing', like a heavy weight on the chest, which may radiate up into the neck or down into the left arm.

It is necessary to stress – at the risk of making some readers neurotic about every twinge they get in the chest – that angina can be misinterpreted. Thus, pressure on the nerves in the neck can radiate down the arm like 'pins and needles', alternatively, especially if the pain comes on after a meal, it can be put down to indigestion. Thirdly, if the pain occurs at night, heartburn due to acid reflux up from the stomach into the oesophagus may be blamed. The most important clue to distinguishing angina from these other conditions is that it is almost invariably brought on by exertion.

(ii)Abdominal pain: There are two types of abdominal pain in particular whose significance can be overlooked. The first is a boring pain in the pit of the stomach brought on by eating, which may be partially relieved by drinking milk or taking antacids. Most people recognise this immediately as gastritis or a peptic ulcer. If it is just the odd twinge that improves with something bought from the chemist, it can be tempting to rely on self-treatment without bothering to see the doctor. This is probably fair enough for those who have had these symptoms on and off over the years, but if it is new and, particularly if it is associated with occasional vomiting or loss of interest in food, there is a danger one might be overlooking a large ulcer or a stomach tumour.

The second is a colicky type of pain which arises to a crescendo, eases off and then restarts, which may come on soon after eating and is associated with a change of bowel habits, such as constipation or diarrhoea. The assumption might be that this is just a stomach upset and self-treatment with laxatives or anti diarrhoeal agents is common. However, a stomach upset of this sort should rarely last longer than a week. If symptoms persist beyond this time there is a possibility there might be an obstruction to the colon due to a polyp or tumour.

When equivocal symptoms do turn out to be serious, the patient may feel guilty he did not seek medical attention earlier, or aggrieved the doctor did not find out what was wrong more quickly. Rarely, however, is the delay in diagnosis important.

To be sure, the patient may have suffered for longer than necessary for what turned out to be an eminently treatable condition: aches and pain due to polymyalgia rheumatica, for example, or shortness of breath due to mild heart failure. But once treatment has been started, the perhaps unnecessarily prolonged period of disability is soon forgotten and no harm is done.

It is more problematic when the equivocal symptom turns out to be cancer. It is natural to feel that "if only I had acted sooner" it might have been caught earlier, and be more easily treatable. But again, delay rarely makes much difference, as by the time a tumour causes symptoms, it has already been growing for several years. This means one of two things. If it is found to be localised and so readily curable by radio-therapy or an operation, then a delay of a month or two does not matter. If, on the other hand, it has already spread, then the likelihood is that this occurred well before the first onset of symptoms, so an earlier diagnosis would not have changed matters.

Nonetheless, there are five symptoms where a delay in diagnosis is definitely undesirable. Some have already been mentioned, but there is no harm in reiterating them.

- Many people perhaps surprisingly ignore *sudden transient paralysis or blindness*, keeping their fingers crossed, hoping it will not happen again. It usually means that a small clot or embolus has passed down one of the arteries to the brain or the retina at the back of the eye and later dispersed. This is an early warning sign of a stroke which, if treated with blood-thinning drugs, may be averted.

- When *acute pain in the eye* is accompanied by blurring of vision and haloes around lights after sitting in the dark for some time – say while in the cinema or watching television – this is an early symptom of acute glaucoma or raised pressure within the eyeball, which can be prevented by medical treatment.
- If *an acute tender headache (temporal arteritis)* is not treated promptly with steroids, blindness may result.
- This early symptoms of a heart attack – *heaviness or pain in the chest, usually brought on by exertion* – are mentioned again to emphasise how they may be misinterpreted as being due to neuralgia, indigestion or heartburn. Prompt attention saves lives.
- *Hoarseness* which does not improve after a couple of weeks may be the first symptoms of a tumour of the larynx which, too, is readily curable in its early stages.

5

SORTING THINGS OUT

Sorting things out, or how doctors make a diagnosis, is the tricky part of medicine. How is it that when you visit the doctor complaining of, say, chest pain, he almost blithely dismisses nine out of ten possible causes to plump for the right one?

Most of the time it is staggeringly obvious what is going on. Indeed, it is not unusual for a patient to tell their doctor what is the matter, as in "I think I must have an ulcer" or "My sciatica is playing up again". The art of diagnosis really only applies to difficult cases, at which point it gets interesting but is almost impossible to describe, requiring as much intuition as experience.

It can be helpful, however, to illustrate the logical steps that lead up to a diagnosis, and particularly to distinguish between the different approaches adopted by general practitioners and hospital specialists.

The family doctor's main concern is to pick out from the tide of problems that pass through his surgery every day the ones that might be serious, whose causes need to be clarified and which may need to be referred onward for a specialist opinion. This is not necessarily easy. The specialist's responsibility, by contrast, is to make a definitive diagnosis and define it accurately enough so that the best treatment can be decided on.

If we return to the three broad categories of illness mentioned in the previous chapter, it is possible to examine how things are sorted out.

In acute-serious illnesses – nasty infections, a heart attack or stroke – it is obvious what is happening, or if not, at least that the patient is ill and needs to be admitted to hospital. Chronic-degenerative diseases – blurring of vision due to cataracts, loss of mobility to arthritis, difficulty of urination due to an enlarged prostate and so on – are also usually fairly obvious. The difficulty comes, yet again, with our third group, the equivocal symptoms. Is a minor problem such as constipation just constipation? Are aches and pains just 'getting on', or the signs of a treatable such as like polymyalgia? Is tiredness, just tiredness or the first symptom of an underactive thyroid?

Here the doctor instinctively applies the three cardinal criteria we have already come across for distinguishing the serious from the non-serious: is it a new symptom? Has it lasted longer than it should? And is it getting worse? If the answer to one or more of these is 'yes', then the three strands of the diagnostic process are evoked to elucidate what is going on. They are a 'history' of the complaint, the physical examination and, where necessary, investigation. We can follow this process by considering the case of Mrs Julie Lock as mentioned in the last chapter, who used to be very active on the local council, but now feels 'tired all the time' and wonders how she ever found the energy to lead such a busy life. Is Mrs Lock's tiredness 'psychological' or the first symptom of a physical illness?

1. The History

The history is the most important part of diagnosis, providing the answer in virtually all cases. The doctor, by asking *exactly* what is complained of, what brings it on, and what relieves it, gets his patient to draw a metaphorical picture of what is happening which, with the help of years of experience, allows him to recognise a typical pattern of symptoms. So, what type of tiredness is Mrs Lock complaining of? Is it of long duration (much more likely to be psychological), or of recent onset (more likely to be physical)? Are there associated symptoms of depressive illness (difficulty in sleeping, irritability) or those that might point to a physical cause (loss of weight, loss of appetite, night sweats, etc.)?

2. The Physical Examination

During the physical examination, the doctor systematically examines the heart, lungs and abdomen while looking for signs of illness such as weight loss, pallor or enlarged lymph nodes that might suggest a physical cause of tiredness.

3. Investigations

When the diagnosis remains in doubt, the doctor will often suggest a range of investigations in the hope that something might turn up, starting with a full blood count (FBC) and ESR (erythrocyte sedimenatation rate which measures the speed with which a column of blood cells [erythrocytes] settles over an hour). These two very simple tests are immensely useful as a mild anaemia and a markedly raised ESR (usually more than 50) are strongly suggestive of something serious. Further than this, a chest X-ray and blood tests, assessing the function of the liver, kidneys, thyroid and the blood sugar, may, albeit infrequently, turn up some unexpected abnormalities.

The process of making a diagnosis is sometimes compared to the work of a detective following up clues, in relentless pursuit of 'the truth'. Much more frequently, the patient tells the doctor the diagnosis, or rather if the doctor listens carefully and shrewdly enough and asks the right questions, the cause presents itself. The more complex and obscure the symptom, the more significant the history becomes; so eliciting that Mrs Lock's tiredness is present the whole time, and that nothing makes it better, when combined with a normal physical examination and normal investigations, suggests it is almost certainly due to a psychological disorder such as depression.

When the general practitioner is foxed, or his diagnosis requires further evaluation, it is time for a specialist's opinion. The specialist has to exclude potentially confusing possible diagnoses and decide on the most appropriate treatment. This can be illustrated by considering how he may tackle the problem of a man in his sixties complaining of chest pain, which from the history and examination he has a pretty shrewd idea is probably due to heart disease. How does he proceed from there?

He must first consider other possible causes of pain in the chest – does it derive from the lungs, the spine, the oesophagus or the heart? Though he may suspect the pain is due to heart disease, he needs to exclude these other possible sources. Accordingly, he will proceed to organise one or more of the following investigations:

- *a chest X-ray* to see if there is any abnormality in the lungs

- X-ray of the spine looking for arthritis
- *a barium meal or endoscopy* to inspect the inner lining of the oesophagus to see whether excess acidity or a hiatus hernia might be contributory factors.

If all these tests turn out to be normal, then he will focus his attention on the heart to find out as much as possible about how it is functioning. This involves:

- *an electrocardiogram (ECG)* or heart reading
- *an echocardiogram* which looks at the functioning of the valves and the movement of the heart wall
- *a coronary angiogram* A catheter is passed from the groin into the arteries to the heart through which a dye is injected that will show the degree of narrowing.

This may all sound a bit pedantic and indeed it is wrong to suggest investigations necessarily follow this logical pattern. The example does, however, illustrate the purpose of the specialist investigation. Obviously the intention is to make a diagnosis, but it is more than that. Other possibilities that might be exacerbating the symptoms or even mimicking them must be included. Thus, if the barium x-ray showed a reflux of acid up the oesophagus, this would mean our sixty-year-old patient really had two causes of his chest pain – both heart disease and heartburn.

Then, thorough investigation is a prerequisite of appropriate treatment. The angiogram might show a narrowing of the coronary artery, which is readily amenable to dilation by a balloon, or some form of bypass surgery. Alternatively, it might show that an operation is *not* possible, which is disappointing for the patient; but at least his symptoms can be tolerated knowing that everything possible has been done.

The good physician will select from the total range of investigations at his disposal those most likely to produce the most definitive results most promptly. This, however, does not prevent a suspicion that some tests are done just because they can be, rather than to illuminate a diagnostic conundrum.

Here the patient is caught in the trap of not knowing enough to determine how essential any test might be. The question "is it really necessary?" can too easily be brushed off with 'I would not be suggesting it if it were not'. It might be better to enquire discreetly what the test is expected to reveal and how this might influence any subsequent treatment.

Finally, one might well wonder whatever happened to the wise old doctor with his black bag who would walk into the sick room and make an instant diagnosis? It is a good point, and many older physicians fear the subtle art of diagnosis has long been lost in a welter of investigations. The consolation is that they are a requirement for the best of modern medicine. Before it became possible to bypass blocked arteries it was not necessary to visualise them with an angiogram. Now they can be, and the angiogram is as essential as the operation itself.

Diagnostic investigations

Accurate diagnosis boils down to being able to *see* what is happening and there are essentially five ways of doing this.

X-rays
There is no mystery about an X-ray of the chest or foot, but one of the most significant developments of modern medicine is the angiogram, where dye is injected into the artery and X-rays

cont.

---

are taken that beautifully delineate both the blood supply to an organ and the functioning of the organ itself. The commonest indication is heart disease to see whether narrowed arteries might be suitable for dilation (angioplasty) or to be bypassed.

Ultrasound

The ultrasound is a small metal disc which is moved around on the surface of the skin over the abdomen or chest putting out pulsed sound waves which bounce off the organs within. The 'echoes' transmitted back form a picture of their structure. Ultrasound is particularly useful for examining the heart, gall bladder, ovaries and pelvis.

Radioistope scan

The radioisotope is a chemical which has been rendered radioactive, and this is injected into a vein. It travels around the body and depending on which chemical has been used is 'taken up' by abnormal tissues in the thyroid, bone or liver.

Endoscopy

There are few sites left in the body where a skilled endoscopist cannot now pass his fibre-optic scope, through which he can directly visualise the inside of the organ as well as being able to take a bite, or biopsy, for examination later under a microscope. Each type of endoscopy requires a slightly different technique and they are named after the organ which is being looked into. The bronchoscope goes down the bronchial airway, the colonoscope travels round the colon, the cystoscope goes into the bladder and the arthroscope into the joint.

Body scanner

If it is necessary to see everything that is going on (especially in the brain) in hauntingly clear detail then a body scan is what is needed. There are two types: the CT scanner and the MRI scanner.

NHS or Private Medicine?

This chapter has been based on the assumption that the reader will be using the National Health Service, but there is always the option of going private. Those able to afford private medical insurance will certainly have access to a better service – though not necessarily better medicine – and are presumably quite glad to pay for it. The important question is whether those less well off are justified in making the financial sacrifice and if so, what sort of medical insurance they should seek. It is therefore necessary to review what one does (and does not) get for one's money.

There is no justification for having a private family doctor or GP. Private medical insurance will not pay for his or her attention, so all consultations have to be paid out of one's own pocket at considerable expense and prescriptions have to be paid at their full price. Anyhow, general practice in the NHS is generally (though not universally) of high quality. It is worthwhile spending some time and ingenuity finding a good GP. He is the gateway to the services of the specialist and it is remarkable how much he can speed up out-patient appointments or clarify uncertainties if he is prepared to make the effort. It sounds ridiculous, but finding the opportunity to thank your family doctor for sorting out a problem can pay dividends over the years, as he is much more likely to make that extra effort on your behalf.

There are nonetheless three specific advantages of going private, all of which are to do with access to specialist services. The most important is that it shortens the wait either to have a problem sorted out (is the cause of this cough serious? What is the skin rash that puzzles the family doctor?) or to have surgical problems like arthritic hips, cataracts and an enlarged prostate gland operated on promptly.

Secondly, private medical insurance allows the option of seeing the physician or surgeon of your choice rather than the NHS consultant (usually at the local hospital) to whom your GP has referred your problem. This is, for the most part, a spurious advantage. All consultants, whether NHS or private (and almost all practise in both sectors) are trained to a similar level of competence, with only marginal differences of skill or manner between them. The benefit here is not so much 'the consultant of your choice' but rather that he will take a personal interest in your case, have the time to explain what is going on, justify the various tests he proposes and ensure they are done promptly and have time to discuss the treatment. There is little point in pretending this is not a better service than the NHS usually provides, even though in the end the treatment you receive will be exactly the same were you one of the same consultant's NHS patients.

The third advantage of going private is for the hospital amenities of private rooms, telephones, good food and, regrettably, often a better quality of nursing.

These, then, are the three advantages, all useful, but scarcely mandatory. Further, there are crucial qualifications in every private insurance policy about what is not covered. These, obviously, exclude medical problems you already have so if you already have Parkinson's or heart disease you will have to pay for treatment out of your own pocket. Similar exclusions may operate for 'incurable' conditions such as Alzheimer's disease or the final stages of a serious illness such as cancer. Preventive treatment and health checks are not covered, and the drugs have to be paid for at full price. Further, and this will depend on the sort of insurance taken out, it will not necessarily cover the full cost. Some of the cheaper policies have a maximum limit, so if you need an operation which comes in over the top you might well end up having to find the difference yourself.

What all this means is that private insurance covers the treatment of acute illnesses or well-defined surgical conditions, but beyond that, many have no alternative other than to rely on the NHS.

There are several competitive policies to choose from, depending on whether you wish to be treated at one of the teaching hospitals or some smaller hospital in the suburbs. The fees are also stratified according to age. Those whose main reason for seeking private health care is to avoid waiting for their operations can opt to pay a much lower premium on the basis that if the NHS waiting list is greater than a defined time for their condition, they can have it done privately. The truth is that to provide comprehensive insurance against all the medical problems one might encounter over the age of sixty is not a reasonable possibility for insurance companies, so for those who cannot readily afford it the medical insurance options are necessarily limited.

At the end of sorting things out, it should be possible to attach a label or diagnosis to virtually any symptom. It is rare indeed for the doctor to be left scratching his head as to what is going on. Armed with a diagnosis some might wish to learn more and make tracks for the public library to consult its medical textbooks. The clearest of these is *The Oxford University Textbook of Medicine*, which can be interpreted with the help of *Black's Medical Dictionary*. It describes the causes (where known), the pattern of the disease, how it presents and what the complications might be. Alternatively, for those who are wired up to the Internet, an hour or two spent surfing will almost invariably generate reams of information about their condition.

6

PUTTING THINGS RIGHT

To do nothing is also a good remedy.
Hippocrates, *Aphorisms I*

Much the best of treatments is nothing at all: the best prescription is the friendly reassurance that whatever ails you is passing, it is not necessary to swallow pills to make it better, while a bit of stoicism and a few days' rest in bed is all that is needed.

Some doctors are very keen on doing nothing. They are therapeutic minimalists instinctively suspicious of the claims for 'wonder' drugs and aware that all remedies can have adverse side-effects. They put their trust in the body's ability to heal itself. Certainly for every ill, no matter how insignificant, there is a pill, and the harm caused by over-treatment is certainly much greater than any caused by under-treatment.

There are variations on the principle of 'the best treatment is no treatment'. One is to advise something fairly innocuous – like an antacid for an episode of gastritis – knowing there are more potent remedies in reserve if this does not do the trick. Alternatively, there is the 'wait and see' option. A joint replacement will certainly get rid of the pain of an arthritic hip, but it might be best to see if it just improves (as it sometimes can) or until the symptoms become so severe it is apparent to all that there really is no alternative.

In Britain, this essentially conservative attitude is much commoner than, for example, the United States or Western Europe, where most patients are treated privately and there is every incentive for doctors to start patients quickly on treatment. It can, however, be overdone and regrettably some patients suffer unnecessarily because their doctors fail to treat their pain or insomnia or indigestion with potent enough remedies. It is not possible to give specific advice here other than to alert readers to what is going on – why the treatment they receive may be so different and so much more or less effective than that of an acquaintance with a similar complaint.

It is not just doctors but their patients whose attitudes range from the minimalist to the interventionist. Some people make a virtue out of 'never being one to take pills' (almost everyone claims to fall into this category), while others prefer to take everything that is available. Similarly with surgery; one person might be so fearful of operations he puts it off till the last moment, while another might argue, "my painful hip makes me so miserable, I can only just get round nine holes of golf at the weekend. I want an operation now."

For those whose treatment fails to alleviate their symptoms, there is always the option of asking the doctor for something a bit stronger. This is best done tactfully – not "the drugs you gave me were useless", as this can be interpreted as a criticism of his competence. Alternatively, for those who are sceptical about a proposed course of treatment, the question "do I have to take it?" can precipitate the brush-off "I wouldn't be suggesting it if not". Asking rather "what will happen if I don't take the treatment?" signals that you wish to discuss the various options in more detail.

It is now time to turn to the various ways in which medicine can put things right with Drugs, Surgery and The Alternatives.

Drugs

Bernard Shaw famously described medicine as "doctors prescribing drugs of which they know little for patients of whom they know less". It is certainly entirely reasonable to ask how doctors can ever be familiar with the 4000 drugs to be found in a modern textbook of therapeutics. They are not. Rather, they will have a shortlist of perhaps twenty drugs which they know well and which they rarely wander outside – a couple of antibiotics, a favourite anti-inflammatory drug, an antidepressant, a sleeping pill and so on.

The apparent cornucopia of drugs conceals the fact that most are either a slight variation of one chemical, or the same chemical under a different name. Each drug has its own chemical (or *generic*) name while the pharmaceutical company gives it its own *proprietary* name. Drug companies spend a lot of money trying to differentiate their own brand from others, but to all intents and purposes the differences tend to be negligible.

Nonetheless, the possibility of moving outside the best tried remedies remains important. Not everyone with raised blood pressure will respond to the standard treatment such as a betablocker, or it may cause unacceptable side-effects such as lethargy or tiredness. There is, then, the option of either trying a different variation of the same drug (ringing the changes), finding another drug to work with it, or changing to a different type altogether.

To be sure, there is little one can do to influence which drug is prescribed, but it is important to ensure it is prescribed in the form that is easiest to comply with. There are, after all, many reasons why people may fail to take their medication as is well illustrated by the example of raised blood pressure (or hypertension).

First, hypertension has no symptoms, so the pills are being taken to reduce the risk of a stroke at some indefinite time in the future, which may or may not happen. Then, once started, treatment must be continued indefinitely, which encourages one to think that if these pills have to be taken for fifteen years or more, it does not matter much if one misses the occasional dose. Thirdly, it may be necessary to take more than one type of drug to lower the blood pressure effectively. Finally, and most importantly, the drug may have subtle side-effects, insufficient perhaps to stop taking them altogether but enough to take the skip out of your step.

Since there are so many reasons for not complying with the doctor's medication, every drug should be given in the form that is easiest to take. Thus, a patient with raised blood pressure can be treated most cheaply with a *generic* form of a betablocker like Propranolol which does not stay long in the bloodstream and so has to be taken three times a day. It is much simpler to take a long-acting *proprietary* form like Inderal LA, which only needs one dose in the morning. If this by itself is insufficient to control blood pressure and another drug such as a water pill or diuretic has to be taken in addition, the simplest solution is a combined preparation of the two. Clearly, taking a single, albeit more expensive, *proprietary* long-acting and combined drug is a lot easier than having to take two or more *generic* drugs several times a day.

It is not unusual for people to complain that they don't want to have to carry on taking drugs – like those for hypertension – for years. They want something to cure the problem in the first place, but this is to misunderstand the nature of modern therapeutics. There are, in fact, very few curative drugs (antibiotics for infections being an obvious example), rather the purpose of most medication is to correct or palliate those chronic, degenerative conditions associated with 'getting on' and for which there is no magic cure. These might be to alleviate aches and pains, cramps or insomnia, which can be mitigated by taking an occasional pill to relieve them in much the same way that one might take an aspirin during an attack of flu. These are summarised in the box below.

Box 1: Take a Pill – Drugs that counteract the symptoms of 'getting on'

Forgetfulness: The simple forgetfulness that is common past the age of fifty often elicits the wry observation "I must be going senile", though by itself it bears no relationship to senility. There is regrettably no magic drug to improve memory, though nicotine appears to stimulate neurotransmitters in the brain and has been shown to improve concentration and intellectual function generally. Nicotine is obviously readily available from the local tobacconist, but those who have given up smoking might try taking nicotine in the form of chewing gum, a patch or as a spray.

Insomnia: Insomnia is a curse of 'getting on' and can lead to chronic exhaustion. Those who would like a good night's sleep and don't mind taking sleeping pills should have no hesitation in asking for them. The most commonly prescribed are nitrazepam and temazepam, though if the effect seems to be wearing off it is sometimes useful to switch to a different type, such as zimovane.

cont.

Heartburn: Heartburn is a terrible nuisance, because it inter-feres with a good night's sleep. There are a number of possible remedies. Simple antacids can be useful but it is better to try and reduce the amount of acid secreted by the stomach, which is the underlying cause. The standard treatment here is the drug cimetidine, though in more servere cases where there is inflammation of the lower part of the oesophagus omeprazole is probably better. When heartburn is associated with a hiatus hernia and the symptoms do not respond to these forms of treatment, then an operation to repair the hernia may be considered.

Night cramps: Night cramps can be prevented by taking quinine sulphate at night or one of a variety of possible alternative remedies, including putting magnets or corks in the mattress.

Aches and pains: There are many causes of aches and pains which, if chronic or persistent, need to be elucidated. But when the complaint is relatively mild, then simple treatment is called for. This takes two forms. Standard analgesics such as para-cetamol and aspirin often provide relief, although they work better when combined with codeine as in coproxamol or solpadol. These can be taken two at a time to a maximum of eight a day. Next, there is a vast range of anti-inflammatory drugs some of which, like Nurofen, can be bought over the counter, though the stronger ones like indomethacin and voltarol are only available on prescription. Some are now available in the form of a topical application which can be applied on the site of maximum tenderness, from where they are absorbed through the skin.

Alternatively, the condition may be more serious or persistent, but again the only option is to take the medication that modifies, limits or suppresses the symptoms. Thus, pain killers or anti-inflammatory drugs may be the only way of controlling the discomfort of arthritis while preventive drug treatment for raised blood pressure must also – as discussed – be taken indefinitely. Obviously, this long-term treatment is not to be started lightly and should be reviewed at regular intervals to ensure that one is on the best possible group of drugs and at the right dosage.

Side-Effects

The need for long-term medication by definition increases the likelihood of side-effects – a matter of considerable, indeed probably disproportionate, importance to many, which necessarily requires some clarification. Most people taking drugs have few, if any, side-effects. There would be no modern pharmaceutical industry if their products were so distressing that whatever benefit they might have were outweighed by the toxic effects they produce. The corollary, however, is equally true – if a compound is biologically active it will have some side-effects in some people. Only useless drugs have no side-effects. So to argue against the use of a drug because it might have side-effects is irrational. If an illness is worth treating, then it must carry the risk that the treatment might be injurious to some.

Several different types of side-effect can be distinguished. First are those that may occur with virtually any drug – rashes, nausea, vomiting and diarrhoea, headaches and so on. Next there are the almost inevitable side-effects which are a consequence of the therapeutic effect the drug attempts to achieve. Thus, insomniacs who take sleeping tablets to help them through the night should not be surprised if the following morning they feel a bit drowsy. Then there are the side-effects which are common (i.e. occuring in one in ten or more of those taking them) associated with a particular type of drug and which are due to its mode of action. Betablockers for the treatment of raised blood pressure also lower the output of blood from the heart, so tiredness and cold extremities are common; antidepressants will, by increasing the activity of certain chemicals in the brain, cheer you up, but that same action acting on other nerves in the body can cause nausea or a dry mouth. Finally, there are the idiosyncratic side-effects which cannot be predicted, are very rare (occuring in one in 100,000 people) but can be very serious.

Clearly, what one does about these side-effects depends on which category they fall into. Some, especially the minor ones, do become less noticeable with time, so it is best to persevere. For others, there is not much that can be done – if depression is severe enough to warrant treatment, then one just has to put up with the dry mouth or nausea that are associated with some forms of antidepressant. Finally, there is no way of predicting the few who might experience the potentially catastrophic idiosyncratic side-effects.

It is difficult to advise as to how diligently one should enquire about the side-effects of a drug. It is one thing to learn that a drug may sometimes cause a skin rash as this is maybe perceived as an acceptable risk. However, learning the same drug may, albeit rarely, cause liver failure could be sufficiently disheartening for a patient to refuse treatment. It is sensible to ask, "what are the *common* side-effects?"

The best source of information about drugs is the *British National Formulary* which is available through most book-shops. It is a bit technical, but useful not just for the information it contains but because it is written by experts who give their opinion on the best treatment for any condition. For those who might be bothered to do so, this gives the opportunity to check your doctor's treatment against expert opinion. So, for raised blood pressure it lists in order the appropriate drugs, starting with the simplest and best tried. Then there are the Cautions – circumstances in which drugs should be prescribed with care. Next are the Contraindications – those medical conditions for which drugs should definitely not be prescribed. Finally there are the Side-Effects – but only the common ones are given so if something you think may be due to the drugs is not listed, that should not discourage you from reporting it.

Surgery

The scope of surgery has shifted dramatically over the last twenty-five years, away from the task of saving lives to alleviating the physical discomforts of 'getting on'. This may be 'spare-part' surgery: if cataracts are clouding your vision, whip them out and insert a plastic lens. Why hobble painfully around the golf course when ten days in hospital will give you a new hip? Or it may be surgery to relieve some anatomical obstruction like an enlarged prostate or blocked artery.

Sooner or later it will be suggested that you might benefit from one or more of these procedures, which raises an interesting set of questions. The intention is to relieve symptoms rather than to save life, so it is natural to prevaricate over whether to take up the option, or to wonder how bad the symptoms have to be before the probability of relieving them outweighs the small risk of any operation.

These 'running repair' type operations are summarised

below and so here I will limit the discussion to the advantages and risks of surgery, how to prepare for it and what to expect afterwards.

The pros and cons of surgery are best considered by asking the question "is my operation really necessary?" The answer is, needless to say, relative. There is no absolute necessity for having a painful hip replaced or cloudy cataract removed. The late Malcolm Muggeridge maintained that the deterioration of his eyesight in later life had allowed him to turn his back on 'earthly vanities' and concentrate instead on his 'inner vision', and so he had no intention of having his cataracts operated on.

There is thus a strong element of personal choice and inclination. Should an arthritic golfer have a joint replacement when he is no longer able to get round eighteen holes; or should it be nine holes, or even three? It will depend essentially on how fanatical he is about golf. The decision, of course, is not entirely yours. Surgeons are reluctant to undertake surgery unless there is sufficient misery to warrant it – for two reasons. Firstly, there is always the possibility that the operation might render the patient worse off than before. Thus, an operation such as a hip replacement may technically be very successful but if, as happens occasionally, it is complicated by a wound infection, the presence of the spare part impedes the body's natural healing process and can be very difficult to deal with. In some cases, it may be necessary to remove the new joint altogether so the patient, instead of having a moderately painful hip now has a stiff and immobile leg. This disappointment can be very difficult for both patient and surgeon to deal with, and to render this type of complication in any way acceptable there has to be the feeling that there was sufficient reason for the operation in the first place.

In the United States, where there are so many surgeons who

all have to make their living, there is little doubt that hips and cataracts are often replaced long before it is necessary. In Britain, by contrast, waiting lists are long enough to ensure that by the time a patient gets to the top he really does need his operation.

Thus, the likelihood of being ill-advised to have surgery in Britain is slender. The problem is exactly the reverse – there are far too many people sitting on waiting lists up and down the country who would benefit considerably from 'running repair' type operations, but who must wait their turn and suffer in silence.

Most of this type of surgery is straightforward. The indications are clear-cut, the procedures well established, good recovery is almost guaranteed while the decision to turn down an operation will not have disastrous consequences. A different set of considerations apply when the question "is my operation really necessary?" applies to 'heroic' surgery for heart disease and cancer. These will be clarified in more detail in the relevant chapters later on but it is useful to consider some principles here.

Surgical Dilemmas

The dilemma of operating on the heart (and essentially this means coronary bypass surgery) is that the greater the need for the operation (i.e. the more severe the heart disease), the greater the risk of some severe complication during or after the operation. Coronary bypass surgery rarely prolongs life, though it is very good at relieving the symptoms of anginal pain. The problem, then, is, at what stage are those symptoms sufficiently severe to risk an operation that might dramatically improve them, but which could prove lethal? Here it is very important to be guided by the surgeon's advice. He is unlikely to recommend surgery unless there is an even chance that the benefits will be considerable; and once again there is the protection, in Britain, that the long waiting lists means they are unlikely to be undertaken lightly. The major concern with cancer surgery is whether it makes a lot of difference to the final outcome. People are obviously prepared to undergo major operations in the hope that the malignancy can be removed. The drawback is that if this is not possible (because it has spread too far), then on top of all the problems of coping with the cancer itself, comes the pain and misery of recovering from a major operation. This risk has certainly diminished in recent years, as scans and X-rays can accurately assess the degree of spread and so the operability of any tumour. Nonetheless, it is fair to say that some surgeons are perhaps more keen to operate than others, and if in doubt it is sensible to seek a second opinion.

The serious risks of all types of surgery increase with age, so a patient's physical condition might disqualify him from having an operation. Of course, if you search hard enough, and certainly if you are prepared to go privately, it is almost always possible to find a surgeon prepared to take that risk on your behalf. Nonetheless, in most circumstances if the verdict is that the risk is too great, then that should be lived with. There is always the possibility that a surgeon may advise against an operation or refuse to perform it simply because it is technically more difficult than he can cope with, or because he feels he has more deserving cases which take priority. This seems unlikely, but if there appears to be no specific reason why an operation is advised against in someone who is otherwise healthy for their age, then again a further opinion should be obtained.

It probably makes little difference which surgeon performs

the operation. There are some with magic fingers whose operations invariably turn out well and certainly in the more rarified forms of surgery there are some who might be seen as better than others. But the long years of surgical apprenticeship and the difficulty of getting to the top results in an extremely high general level of competence. Even the most complex operations become routine with practice, and the outcome is much more likely to be influenced by the patient's physical well-being and the quality of care in the immediate aftermath.

This is a good thing, because there is very little personal choice in the matter. The decision of who does the operation is essentially determined by your GP who, except in unusual circumstances, will refer you to a specialist at the local hospital. Of course if the operation is to be done privately, then there is the possibility of choosing your surgeon, but this is no less arbitrary as there is no guarantee that he or she will be any more or less competent than the surgeon at your local hospital. If there is any advice to be given about choosing one's surgeon, it is to be slightly wary of the distinguished surgeon approaching the end of his career with a considerable reputation. The hard-working surgeon in his middle years is most likely to produce the best results.

Preparing for an Operation

The prospect of an operation is certainly not helped by the lack of privacy and impersonality of hospital life. This can be very tedious, especially for those who have slept soundly in their own beds for forty years. It is important to take along a few personal pleasures to cheer you up and, outside the privileged world of private hospitals where there is sometimes very good food, a decent bottle of wine and something special from the delicatessen are essential. Earplugs are a must and a Sony Walkman recommended.

The main fear of surgery is the pain and discomfort that follows an operation – lying on an operating table for several hours while a surgeon inflicts major wounds is severely stressful. To minimise this, it is important to be as fit as possible. It is a suitable opportunity for smokers to quit, and for those who do not take regular exercise a brisk walk for an hour a couple of times a day is mandatory. The anaesthetist will decide if you are fit for surgery, but as this assessment usually does not happen until just before the operation, it is sensible to visit your own doctor in advance to have your blood pressure checked and to treat vigorously any illness such as a chest infection with antibiotics. It is very frustrating to go into hospital only to have the operation cancelled on medical grounds.

The anxiety preceding an operation is mitigated by an injection of a tranquilliser and the journey to the operating theatre usually takes place under a mellow haze. It also induces amnesia, so the following day little is remembered of the ordeal. There is, however, something of a conspiracy of silence about the pain following an operation. Patients realise it will hurt afterwards and are ashamed to express their fears, while the surgeon and anaesthetist, knowing it will be bearable, do not volunteer false reassurances. As one anaesthetist rather gloomily puts it: "The ideal drug has not yet been discovered to relieve satisfactorily either severe or moderate pain." The dilemma is that the more potent the pain-relieving drug, the more likely it is either to depress the respiration or have other unwanted side-effects such as nausea or confusion. The standard procedure is therefore to give painkillers on a regular basis rather than when they are asked for, the intention being to keep a steady level of the drug in the tissues to stop pain breaking through.

Besides pain, most patients will experience one or other 'minor' complications of anaesthesia – called minor not because they are trivial, indeed they are not, but to distinguish them from serious problems like a stroke or heart attack. Thus, about a third of patients will suffer nausea and vomiting, although interestingly this decreases with age. This is influenced by many factors, such as the type of anaesthetic and painkillers used and the site of the operation – occurring most commonly after operations on the eye, back and abdomen.

Two-thirds of patients come round from the anaesthetic with a sore throat which is due to the minor trauma from the tube that connects them up to the ventilation machine. This is made worse by the drugs used in the induction of anaesthesia that dry up the mucous membranes and by the breathing in of dry anaesthetic gases.

Headache is a common complaint, as is constipation, a combination of too little to eat, physical inactivity and the painkilling drugs which reduce the motility of the gut. Finally, anaesthetics knock you out for much longer than the time spent on the operating table. There is a generalised feeling of weakness and malaise that can last for a month or more.

There may be more serious complications – chest and wound infections, a confusional state and heart problems – but it is reassuring to learn that these occur in less than one in four patients. There is a small chance of a fatal outcome due to the stress of the operation, but this is considerably less than one per cent.

The consolation for all this immediate misery is that it is often obscured by the dramatic relief of the symptoms for which the operation was undertaken. There is no greater thrill for the orthopaedic surgeon than to see someone who had been severely limited by the pain of an arthritic hip walking around the ward a few days after the operation.

Box 2: Running Repairs: What Surgery Offers

Face-lifts: There are three main face-lift operations: to smooth out the forehead, correct bags under the eyes and, the commonest, to restore a firm jaw line. First, the skin is lifted off, any slackness in the underlying muscles is tightened with stitches and then, after trimming, the skin is sewn back in position.

Cataract: The commonest treatable reason for deteriorating eye sight is this murky frosting of the lens. This can be corrected by removing the lens and replacing it with a plastic intraocular [within the eye] lens implant.

Coronary bypass graft: The most effective remedy for the disabling chest pain of angina due to narrowing of the arteries to the heart is to bypass the obstruction with a graft, usually taken from the leg. This connects the aorta (the main artery that runs out of the heart) to the coronary artery beyond the obstruction thus restoring the free flow of blood to the heart muscle and curing the angina.

Pacemaker: A pacemaker may be necessary when the conduction of nerve impulses down in the back of the heart is impaired, leading to slowing of the heart rate or indeed its temporary cessation, resulting in symptoms of tiredness or fainting. A pacemaker 'box' is inserted under the skin on the left side of the chest from which an electrical wire runs to the heart, which takes over the initiation of the contraction of heart muscle.

cont.

Abdominal aneurysm: The abdominal aorta is the conduit through which blood travels from the heart to the leg. If its wall is weakened it will balloon out to form an aneurysm, which may leak with potentially catastrophic consequences. It is advisable that this weakened section be replaced with a teflon graft.

Prostate: The increase in size of the prostate gland that occurs with age obstructs the flow of urine from the bladder, resulting in difficulty in initiating urination and a poor stream. Through a cystoscope passed up the urethra, the surgeon chips away at the gland thus 'reboring' the urethra. This is called a transurethral prostatectomy (TUR).

Stress incontinence: The trauma of childbirth weakens the muscles of the pelvis, including those that act as an external sphincter controlling the flow of urine from the bladder down the urethra. This results in stress incontinence which can be corrected with a variety of operations.

Joint replacement: The hips and knees, the major weight-bearing joints, are prone to arthritis, which can be cured by a joint replacement. These immensely successful operations can restore virtually normal mobility.

The 'Alternatives'

Sooner or later, virtually everyone wonders whether they might not be helped by alternative medicine. This is often inspired by a friend's anecdotal recommendation of some practitioner who, if he has a successful reputation, is to be found in Harley Street, but if not practises from a Victorian terraced house in the suburbs. He has done wonders for a back, or a nagging hip pain or some poorly defined symptom that ordinary doctors could do nothing about. There is no reason for those reporting this to be deliberately misleading, so whether the remedy was acupuncture, osteopathy, herbalism or homeopathy, or any of the other types of alternatives, it did something. The question is what? The antipathy to, or more usually lack of interest in, alternative medicine by mainstream doctors is sometimes misinterpreted as fear of a challenge to their omniscience. But this must be fairly unusual.

There are three more likely reasons. Doctors do not, on the whole, understand the principle behind alternative therapies, mainly because they have never got round to finding out about them. Further, doctors know the training requirements of their own profession and the qualifications of the specialists to whom they refer their patients. It is much more difficult to determine the competence of alternative practitioners, of whom there must be, just as in orthodox medicine, good and bad – anyone, after all, can put up their plaque and become a self-appointed practitioner of naturopathy or herbalism. Finally, there are relatively few scientific evaluations where the claims of alternative medicine to cure serious illnesses have been compared with the results of orthodox medicine.

These are important reservations, so if your doctor appears to be unhelpful there are good reasons for it. It also means that if you are interested in seeking help from alternative medicine, you are very much on your own.

It is actually quite difficult to judge the benefits of the alternatives, though two general points can be made. Alternative, or as they prefer to describe themselves, complementary, practitioners commonly invoke spurious causes for illnesses. Ask any doctor why you have raised blood pressure, diabetes or osteoarthritis, and in all honesty he will shrug his shoulders and say he does not know. These illnesses might be commoner as one gets older, so ageing obviously plays a role. But why one person out of many should have raised blood pressure is almost impossible to say.

Alternative practitioners are more prepared to claim to know the 'cause' which often involves identifying some aspect of the environment, the commonest being the food one eats, pollution or stress. This is beguiling, but not borne out by scientific enquiry.

Then the ways in which treatments are supposed to work often seem to have little or no basis in biology. Acupuncturists will acknowledge that the channels along which they insert their needles are invisible. Homeopaths claim that the more dilute the remedy the more potent it becomes, which would seem to contradict elementary laws of biology.

Yet one is struck with the fact that very often the alternative medicines do seem to work, at least for some people for some illnesses. It is scarcely sensible to pass up the opportunity for help just because there is no good explanation of why it should be successful. What is perhaps suspicious is the way in which different types of alternative medical practitioners claim to be able to treat virtually anything with their own brand of remedy. Thus, something as straightforward as hayfever due to pollen allergy is treated by acupuncturists with their needles, herbalists with their remedies, naturopaths with their dietary recommendations and chiropractors by manipulating the spine. This therapeutic optimism is at least attractive, and certainly preferable to the disillusioned family doctor who has begun to doubt whether anything he does is of any value.

It seems fair, then, to make the following judgments: manipulation whether by osteopaths or chiropractors is known to be of considerable value for those with acute and sometimes chronic back pain and other pains of the joints. Acupuncture offers relief for many forms of pain both acute and intractable, though it is unclear how long the effect lasts. Herbal remedies might well work sometimes – many modern medicines are, after all, based on nothing more than the empirical observation of the therapeutic properties of herbs – indeed, the first major advance in modern therapeutics was the isolation of the heart drug digoxin from the foxglove.

It would, however, seem sensible before seeking help from alternative therapists to try and obtain a specific diagnosis from your own doctor, as diagnosis is not their strongest point. If orthodox treatment is unsatisfactory or ineffective, there is every reason to see whether the alternative practitioner can do better.

When Things Go Wrong: Conclusions

Here are some general observations to conclude this survey in the ways in which medicine seeks to put things right. Some people seem content to put up with medical problems for which others seek medical attention. If this arises from stoicism or general antipathy to taking pills or having operations, fair enough. There seems little point in being virtuous about it.

Modern medicine is highly effective and one should not be put off seeking its aid out of fear that it might do more harm than good. My impression is that many people do not seek medical help often enough, or if they do, they find it insufficiently effective – which brings me to the second point.

The criterion of whether a treatment is working is if it minimises or eradicates the symptoms it sets out to alleviate. If it does not, it is important to know why. To be sure, there may come a time when there is nothing more to do and you simply have to put up with whatever ails you. But before that point is reached, one has to be certain that the best drugs are being given in the best combinations and at the highest tolerable dosage. Similarly, for those conditions amenable to surgery, the possibility of an operation should at least have been discussed.

PART 3

How to Stay . . .

Time flies over us, but leaves its shadow behind.
Nathaniel Hawthorne

Though time flies and the years roll by, how old we feel we are, our 'inner', as opposed to our 'chronological' age, hardly changes and for many of those in their seventh decade or more their enthusiasm, emotions and interests seem much the same as they were forty years earlier. This section examines what can be done when the sparkle of our inner youthful age is compromised by the inevitable physical changes of the passing years, so one can step out of time's shadow and stay – beautiful, perceptive, mobile, cheerful and sexy.

7

BEAUTIFUL

The face, more than any other part of the body, advertises to the world the passage of time. Look down into the stomach or peek inside the abdomen and its appearance is much the same in an eighty-year-old as in an eighteen-year-old, but the face, decade by decade, is a constantly changing landscape, for which there are three reasons.

The first is exposure to the elements. For everyone other than the strictest Muslim, the face is constantly exposed, day-in day-out, to the external elements – pollution, dust and dirt, and particularly the damaging ultraviolet rays of sunlight. Then there is the effect of the muscles of facial expression. There are more separate muscle groups in the face than anywhere else, and for good reason, as they are the means by which we communicate our emotions to one another. Whether smiling, frowning, squinting or looking quizzical, these muscles are constantly moving and in so doing loosen the skin that overlies them. The surface after a while becomes criss-crossed with fine wrinkles. Thirdly, there is the effect of gravity, particularly on the cheeks and under the chin which, with no supporting structures, begin to droop. Compounding all this are the physical effects of ageing itself. When young, the cells on the surface of the face completely renew themselves every eighteen months – and the consequences of the loss of this capacity for self-renewal are obvious enough.

The overall effects of time on facial appearance can be summarised by considering its influence on the three separate layers of skin – which can be compared to a wedding cake. On the outside, the icing or *stratum corneum* is the protective layer of firm, dead cells that are continuously being shed and replaced from the layer beneath. With time, this protective layer becomes dryer and more scaly, which can be prevented to a certain degree by the regular application of a moisturising agent. Then there is the marzipan, or *epidermis* which contains the pigment cells that give the skin its colour. Again, with time the epidermis becomes thinner and the pigment cells can both get bigger or smaller – if they both happen at the same time it leads to a sort of piebald appearance. The minuscule blood vessels within the epidermis may leak to form flat bruises known as senile purpura (purple blotches). Beneath the epidermis is the *dermis*, which consists of supportive and elastic fibres and through which run the nerves and small arteries that nourish the skin. This, too, becomes thinner and as the elastic fibres become less elastic, so wrinkles will form.

From all this, one might conclude that the face is unfairly susceptible to the effects of the passage of time and there is thus every reason, especially as the relevant techniques are so sophisticated, to do something about it.

There are essentially three ways of improving the appearance of the face: anti-wrinkling creams, resurfacing and plastic surgery. First, however, it is necessary to emphasise the benefits of prevention. Clearly the face needs to be protected against the depradations of the ultraviolet rays of sunlight. This is best achieved with the regular application of sunscreens with a protective factor of at least 15, together with avoidance of prolonged exposure in the heat of the day. Further, as is well recognised, smoking accelerates the wrinkling process and so yet another very good reason to abjure the habit.

Anti-Wrinkling Cream

The cosmetics industry is forever proclaiming a major new breakthrough in anti-wrinkling cream, but there is really only one – tretinoin – that has reliably shown to be effective. Tretinoin is a derivative of vitamin A and has been used for thirty years to treat a wide variety of skin conditions, including acne and psoriasis. It was discovered to have an anti-wrinkling effect quite accidentally, when a woman being treated for some other skin condition noted that her wrinkles appeared to regress at the same time. Further investigation revealed that tretinoin increased the amount of collagen fibres, stimulated the cells in the dermis and increased blood flow to the skin.

It is remarkable that a compound should have so many diverse effects and it is presumed that tretinoin acts as a rejuvenator, 'switching on' cells that have become tired and inefficient with age. Its effects have been assessed with serial photographs and, according to a study from Italy, it produces 'a more brilliant and glowing skin'.

The technicalities of its use are as follows: tretinoin is rubbed into the wrinkling parts of the skin at night, with the areas around the eyes responding best. Treatment is usually initiated with the lowest dose cream (.025 per cent) every night or every other night. During the first three months, there is some redness, peeling and itching of the skin which can be mini-mised by a special formulation which incorporates an emollient cream. Tretinoin causes an increased sensitivity to the sun and so should be combined with the application of a sunscreen in the morning.

In the first month, a pleasing pink colour and tightening of the skin becomes apparent. After two months, the fine wrinkles tend to fade. After six months, sagging skin around the mouth tightens. The greatest benefit occurs in the first year, after which it should be applied once or twice a week to maintain the positive results. Tretinoin, prescribed as a retin-A, can only be obtained by private prescription as it is not available on the NHS for the treatment of wrinkles.

Resurfacing

The next stage up from anti-wrinkling creams is to 'resurface' the face by burning off the overlying layer – the stratum corneum, and to a lesser degree the epidermis —and allowing new, fresh skin to grow through. This is particularly useful for those with excess pigmentation and multiple fine wrinkles, but will do little for those with heavy redundant skin folds. There are three techniques in common use:

Chemical peel: The surface of the skin can be burnt off with a chemical such as trichloroacetic acid or Phenol. The procedure is as follows. The chemical is applied and the skin is sealed with adhesive tapes and left for a couple of days, during which the eyes and mouth swell up and talking and drinking can be difficult. When the tapes are removed, they take with them the layer of burnt-off skin, leaving a raw and tender surface which is treated with antiseptic cream. The new skin underneath is pink, as if after a nasty attack of sunburn, and is kept moist with appropriate cream. After a couple of weeks, the patient is ready to face the world again, though a sun block cream is necessary as the skin can become very sensitive to sunlight.

Dermabrasion (literally, abrasion of the skin): This involves the mechanical removal of layers of skin with a rotating diamond wheel or brush. A high level of skill and experience is necessary, as bleeding during the procedure makes visualisation of the result of treatment difficult to assess.

Carbon dioxide laser: The use of a high energy carbon dioxide laser is rapidly becoming the most popular form of resurfacing. The amount of heat-related damage is minimised and very precise removal of thin layers of tissue can be achieved.

These techniques certainly sound quite drastic, so it is useful to quote the judicious opinion of an expert in their use, David A. Sherris, on their benefits and side-effects:

The results of resurfacing can range from disappointing, due to an under-aggressive procedure, to disastrous, due to an over-aggressive one. Nonetheless, well-performed procedures are highly satisfying to patients and physicians alike. Reasonable expectations should include substantial improvement in skin texture and colour as well as the eradication of fine and moderate wrinkles. Severe wrinkles may diminish but usually persist to some degree. Post-operative care may involve the application of full face dressings or ointment and necessitates cleansing numerous times a day. Further, the skin will be fragile, pink and photo-sensitive for weeks to months.

Plastic Surgery

Tretinoin and resurfacing may mitigate fine wrinkles, but will do nothing for the heavy loose folds and furrows on the forehead, baggy eyes and dropping jowls, which are caused by the loosening of the attachment of the skin to the underlying muscles. To correct these, some form of face-lift is required which, starting from the top and working down, will remove the furrows from the forehead, bags from under the eyes (blepharoplasty) and correct drooping of the cheek and jowls.

Forehead lift: The combination of gravity and the loss of elastic tissue can cause deep furrowing of the brow, giving the face a cragged and sometimes angry appearance. The simplest approach is to make an incision along the hairline across the top of the forehead, lift up the skin, dissect away the fat underneath and bring the skin back up taut before resewing it into its new position. For obvious reasons, this technique is not appropriate for those with male pattern baldness where there is no hair to hide the scar. Here a mid-forehead approach is probably more appropriate. Finally, and increasingly popular, is the endoscopic brow lift, which requires no skin excision. Rather, three to six small incisions are made well within the hairline through which an endoscope is introduced, permitting the surgeon to dissect away the redundant skin under direct vision.

Blepharoplasty: It is difficult to appear brilliant and sparkling with drooping eyelids and bags under the eyes. The plastic surgeon corrects the former by a delicate incision, pulling up the eyelid and sewing it into its new position. Correcting bags under the eyes is more complex, as the underlying muscle has to be tightened as well. Following the operation there will be some bruising around the eyes, which is easily concealed with dark glasses but, in the longer term, the lower eyelid may turn outwards, indicating that too much skin has been removed. This may need a further small operation to correct it.

Face-Lift: The commonly used term face-lift is somewhat inaccurate, as it is actually the cheek and neck that are lifted. This is appropriate for those who have downward drooping jowls with excess of skin and laxity of the skin under the chin – commonly referred to as the 'turkey gobbler'. Many different methods have been described, but in broad terms the technique involves the following.

The surgeon starts by making an incision from above and down the front of the ear, then back behind the ear lobe and eventually at right angles into the hairline. The skin is then lifted up and separated off from the underlying muscle, which is cut and lifted upwards and reconnected to the larger neck muscles. The skin is then repositioned, any redundant folds are removed and is just sewn back into position, with a small drain left in place just under the ear to allow any blood or fluid which might be leaking from the disturbed capillaries to drain away. This takes up to three hours. The incision runs most of its path through the hairline, but dark glasses and a discreetly placed scarf over the front of the ear will conceal the scar until it has properly healed.

There are several possible complications. There may be bleeding under the skin, giving rise to a large bruise which is allowed to disperse of its own accord. The wound may break down behind the ear if the skin has been pulled up too tightly and this, too, must be allowed to heal with time. Finally, there is the danger of damage to the nerve fibres under the skin. The sides of the face may be numb for up to twelve months and as the nerves reconnect there may be an unpleasant sensation, rather like ants crawling up the skin. More seriously, but very rarely, the motor nerves and muscles may be bruised, causing the side of the face to droop, though this too should recover with time.

The operation makes a person look fitter and younger, as if just back from a long refreshing holiday. The best effect is a clearer jaw line due to elimination of drooping folds of skin. It is apparently rare to be embarrassed by friends saying "My God, you've had a face-lift," (though this might be because they are naturally tactful).

A face-lift and the other procedures described here are really the only way of restoring the loss of handsome features due to drooping of the skin. The main apprehension for those contemplating an operation is the fear they might fall into the hands of a 'cowboy' plastic surgeon, whose competence they cannot judge and whose results are less than satisfactory. This is certainly a danger in the private clinics that advertise in women's magazines, many of whom do not even offer a pre-operative consultation with the surgeon (or if they do, they charge extra). The only way round this is to ask your general practitioner to arrange for a private referral to one or other of the consultants in a large plastic surgery unit attached to a major hospital. He may not do the operation himself, but will be able to refer you to someone who does. Ethical plastic surgeons are very careful that the rules of good practice are adhered to, and only too aware that their specialist skills can be brought into disrepute by irresponsible elements. They do not advertise, will only take referrals from other doctors and, because their professional reputations are at stake, they take obsessive care with the operation. A few duff face-lifts and a highly lucrative private practice would dry up in no time.

Baldness

There is one thing about baldness – it's neat.

Anon

Balding is an almost universal and completely natural event in males. Nonetheless, the vast range of remedies reported over the last 2500 years reveal a consistent demand for hair restoration. Cleopatra advised the balding Julius Caesar to try a mixture of "ground-up burnt domestic mice, horse teeth, beer grease and deer droppings". The French recommend alcohol and beef fat, the Germans extract of bovine heart and Hungarians horseradish and mustard oil.

There is, not surprisingly, no evidence that any of these unusual remedies are the least bit effective. It has, however, been claimed that increasing the blood flow to the scalp may promote hair growth. Thus the popular medical book *The Household Physician*, published at the turn of the century, advised that baldness might be prevented by "quickening the circulation of the scalp such as by washing the head every morning in cold water, and drying with a rough towel by vigorous rubbing and brushing with a hard brush until the scalp becomes red". Certainly, trauma to the scalp is often followed by regrowth of hair, probably because of the greater blood flow to the injured area. Seeking to capitalise on this effect, the Japanese have reportedly developed a spiky hairbrush with which the bald purchaser is encouraged to strike the head 200 times a day (being a Japanese gadget, the number of strokes is automatically recorded).

The main cause of balding is genetic – that is, the hair follicles are programmed to work for so long and then they pack up in a variety of different patterns. In men this takes the form of a U-shaped recession at the front, combined with baldness over the crown. In women, the frontal hairline is unaffected, but there may be diffuse thinning. Sometimes stress, particularly severe illness and major surgery, may precipitate excess hair loss and very occasionally there may be some underlying condition of the scalp, such as psoriasis, that might be treatable.

The male hormone testosterone plays an important role, as neither those unfortunate enough to be castrated before puberty, nor pseudo-hermaphrodites (who are born genetically male, but whose tissues are insensitive to testosterone and so have the appearance of being female) become bald. One obvious answer to balding men would be to take something that blocks the effect of testosterone, but as this has the disadvantage of promoting breast growth, a squeaky voice and loss of sex drive, it understandably is not a serious prospect.

Medical Treatment

The breakthrough in the medical treatment of baldness was based on the observation by a patient that his scalp became 'hairier', while taking a new blood pressure drug called Minoxidil. The drug manufacturers soon realised this side-effect could be turned to considerable commercial advantage, and Minoxidil was eventually marketed under the splendid name of Regaine as a topical treatment for male pattern baldness. It must be rubbed into the balding scalp twice a day for at least three months before producing any serious hair growth, and once the balding patch has recovered, it must be continued indefinitely, as the new hair has a tendency to fall out.

There is, however, considerable controversy as to how well it works. Studies sponsored by the manufacturers claim that "the majority have subjective hair growth, but few have enough to yield a dramatic cosmetic benefit". Indeed, less than one in ten reported dense hair regrowth which seems a bit disappointing, but the main selling point of Regaine is that it retards or stops balding rather than replacing hair already lost.

The doctor's bible *The Drugs and Therapeutic Bulletin* dismissed Regaine as being suitable "only for the rich and patient". Nonetheless, with 100,000 men in the United States regularly applying it to their scalps, it cannot be completely ineffective.

Hair Transplantation

A hair transplant offers a more realistic method of overcoming baldness. It redistributes what scalp hair remains from the side and back of the head onto the balding dome. It is not an option for those whose balding is far advanced, or when what remains is thin and scanty. As dermatologist Vince Bertucci at the University of Toronto puts it:

The best candidate for hair transplantation is one who has a fine hair texture, large, dense donor sites and who shows minimal contrast between hair and scalp colour. Curly hair maximises the appearance of density. Conversely those with coarse texture, sparse donor site density, extensive baldness and those who show great contrast between scalp and hair shading are unlikely to have good results.

The method is as follows: The 'donor' and 'recipient' areas of the back and top of the scalp respectively are cleansed with antiseptic and infiltrated with local anaesthetic and one or two strips of tissue are harvested from a donor site. Next, the recipient area is prepared by making small incisions in the overlying skin with a punch or scalpel. The grafts are then carefully inserted into these sites and a turban-type pressure dressing is usually applied. Initially, the results may seem disappointing, as the newly transplanted hair promptly falls out, but three months later, when the hair follicles have recuperated, up comes the new head of hair.

An alternative, more difficult, procedure which requires a general anaesthetic is a hair-bearing flap, where a full thickness hair-bearing part of the scalp is skimmed off the back of the head, swivelled round and replaced on the balding pate. This instantly gives a new head of hair, but if it fails the patient will have lost what little hair he had.

Body Contouring

With age comes a major redistribution of the body's fat deposits, which accumulate in the abdominal wall, around the hips and on the inner surface of the thigh. The sensible way to prevent this is a combination of dieting (though the fat in these areas can be remarkably persistent), and regular, twice or three times a week exercise classes with an emphasis on toning the muscles in the abdominal wall and around the buttocks.

Plastic surgery offers the alternative option of body contouring, particularly for those with a drooping apron of fat. Here, a long incision sparing the navel is made up the centre and across the abdomen and the excess fat is freed from the underlying muscle. The skin is then stretched as far as it will go (which sometimes takes it down to the knees) and the redundant folds are cut away. The abdominal muscles are tightened with stitches and everything is sewn back into position leaving an extremely scarred but much tauter tummy. The occasional complications include oozing of blood under the skin which collects as a bruise, and damage to the nerves resulting in numb patches of skin.

Similar principles can be applied to the removal of excess fat from around the buttocks, on the inner thighs and upper arms. The alternative to surgery is liposuction, where a large bore needle is placed under the skin and fat cells are sucked out under pressure.

8

PERCEPTIVE

With time, our precious perceptions of the world around us become gradually less acute. Here we consider the many ways of ensuring we can carry on Seeing, Hearing, Tasting and Smelling.

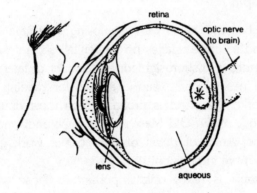

Seeing

The eye is a sublime creation. Light passes through the cornea to be focused by the lens. It then passes through the semiliquid aqueous to fall on the retina, stimulating nervous impulses which travel along the optic nerve into the brain, where the visual message is 'decoded'.

Visual acuity may thus be impaired in one of four ways:

- The lens may become stiffer, losing its ability to focus close images on the retina. This is presbyopia
- The lens may become clouded with a cataract
- The draining of the 'aqueous' may be impaired causing the pressure in the eyeball to rise which can damage the optic nerve. This is glaucoma
- The cells of the retina may deteriorate. This is macular degeneration.

Presbyopia

The lens becomes stiffer with age, losing its ability to change shape and so close images no longer fall accurately on the retina, resulting in short-sightedness. Sooner or later virtually everyone has to start wearing glasses for reading or fine needlework. The effect is probably seen most dramatically in the work of the Old Masters like Rembrandt and Titian, where the clarity of detail of their earlier work gradually becomes more impressionistic in later life.

Presbyopia is really only important in those who, like Jonathan Swift, refuse – through vanity or indolence – to correct it by wearing glasses:

Having by some ridiculous resolution determined never to wear spectacles he could make little use of books in his later years. His ideas therefore not being increased by reading, wore gradually away and left his mind to the vexations of the hour so at last his anger was heightened into madness.

Samuel Johnson

Cataracts

Cataracts, or clouding of the lens, affects virtually everyone over the age of sixty-five, causing haziness or mistiness of vision and glare – where bright lights dazzle and halos may be seen around street lamps.

The yellow discoloration of cataract also absorbs light, thus changing the perception of colour. Violets and blues are the first to be filtered out, until finally only reds can reach the retina. This can clearly be seen in the Impressionist paintings of Monet – a famous cataract sufferer – as he himself observed: "What I painted was more and more dark and when I compared it to my former work, I would be seized by a furious rage and slash at my paintings with a penknife."

The retina compensates by becoming very sensitive to these 'lost colours' so when the cataract is removed the influx of the previously excluded violets and blues overwhelms everything. Returning home after his cataract operation, Monet observed: "The first sensation was of a diffuse blueness, I was surprised at the strange colours of my most recent pictures." He returned to work with enthusiasm, retouching his earlier works until his friends persuaded him to desist. For most people, the effect of cataracts is more mundane – the cloudiness and change in colour perception gives the impression that the house continually needs redecorating.

The only 'cure' for a cataract is to have it removed, but while waiting for an operation the following hints may be helpful:

- The effect of glare can be minimised by wearing a wide-brimmed hat or tinted glasses while outside
- When reading, lighting should be over the shoulder and some find it useful to cover part of the page with a piece of black cardboard to reduce glare from the page.

Most people will wish to defer an operation for as long as possible, though there is no intrinsic advantage in this. The belief that the cataract needs to be 'ripe' before it is plucked is erroneous. Most surgeons prefer to remove one cataract at a time, starting with the worst and dealing with the second a month or two later. The operation is performed under local anaesthetic, administered as a slightly painful injection just under the eyeball. First, the eyelashes are cut to prevent them getting in the way, then the cornea is incised, the lens removed and replaced with a plastic one – an intraocular lens implant. The whole procedure takes about one hour.

In the aftermath two sorts of eyedrops are administered. A combination of antibiotics and steroids will reduce the risk of infection and inflammation respectively, while another type will splint the intraocular lens in place, though temporarily making the eyesight somewhat blurred.

Dr A. E. Clark, consultant physician at the London Hospital, describes his post-operative visual experience:

I can remember the moment to this day. The first thing that struck me was the face and particularly the colours of the pretty nurse. The second was the almost dazzling whiteness of the registrar's white coat. Thirdly it was the brilliant blue of the surgeon's suit and I had always thought he dressed so discreetly. And then I realised the appalling vulgarity and lack of taste of my own multi-coloured striped pyjamas.

The intraocular lens implant will have been chosen to account for the refractive state of the eye before the operation, so far-sight should be near perfect, though short-sight will be impaired and reading glasses are usually necessary. Following surgery, physical activity is restricted till the eye heals after four to six weeks.

Glaucoma

The aqueous fluid within the eye does the same for the eyeball as air does for a football, keeping it round and bouncy. It is constantly being secreted and drains out through the corner of the eye. If this drainage is blocked, the pressure will rise within the eyeball, damaging the optic nerve to cause glaucoma. The loss of vision may be so slow and insidious that most patients only discover they have the condition when the optician measures the pressure within the eyeball with a special machine. They will then notice a 'peripheral' visual defect: whereas a normal-sighted person standing in the middle of the road can see both a car coming towards them and, less distinctly, the figures of pedestrians on the pavement, the person with glaucoma can still see the oncoming car, but is blind to the pedestrians on either side.

Glaucoma needs to be treated, because if the raised pressure within the eyeball is not corrected the loss of peripheral vision will gradually 'close in' to cause total blindnesss.

There are essentially two options. The amount of aqueous fluid can be reduced with drugs or its drainage can be improved with a small operation. It is customary to start with drug treatment, though the results of surgery are so good – controlling the pressure in about 90 per cent of cases – that some eye specialists favour this straight away.

As already discussed, most cases of glaucoma are picked up when people visit their optician to have their glasses changed. For those for whom this is not necessary, it is advisable to have a routine check every few years, and more frequently if there is a history of glaucoma in the family.

Macular Degeneration

Macular degeneration is the most serious of the four visual disorders, as the section of the retina on which the incoming light is focused – the macula – starts to deteriorate. Luckily one eye is usually less affected than the other and for a time the better eye takes over, concealing the visual problem. This starts as a disturbance of the perception of straight lines; then fine visual perception is lost, so it becomes necessary to use some form of magnifying glass or large print books for reading. Whereas glaucoma causes difficulty with peripheral vision, here there are great blobs in the centre of the visual field – making it difficult to see the face of the person with whom one is talking or to get a clear picture of what is on the dinner plate.

Regrettably treatment is not very satisfactory, though there is much hope that a new form of laser therapy may prevent further deterioration. Otherwise, good lighting is essential and low vision aids (LVAs for short) help – the simplest being a magnifying glass or mini telescope which can be carried around in the pocket. Larger magnifying lenses slipped around the neck so they dangle on the chest will allow reading while leaving the hands free. Those severely affected should register as blind. There is little point in stoically holding out against this, especially as the benefits include a reduced television licence fee, and free travel.

Hearing

Oscar Wilde's father, Sir William Wilde, a distinguished ear surgeon in Dublin, once observed in an epigram his son would have been proud of: "There are only two types of deafness – one is due to earwax and is curable. The other is not due to wax [but nerve deafness] and is not curable." This is not strictly true as deafness can also be due to the accumulation of catarrh in the middle ear, otherwise known as glue ear, which reduces the transmission of sound.

Nonetheless, Sir William's distinction is important. Deafness may be conductive, where the passage of sound down the ear canal and its resonance on to the eardrum may be impaired by wax or catarrh respectively, or neural, where the abnormality lies in the auditory nerve and is known as presbyacusis (the loss of hearing associated with ageing).

The correct diagnosis is usually made in the following way. The patient goes to the doctor with 'difficulty in hearing'. The doctor inspects both ears. If these are full of wax then they can be syringed out allowing him to examine the eardrum beyond. This may be inflamed (perhaps due to an infection) or may appear to bulge out due to accumulation of catarrh in the middle ear – usually following a cold. If, despite appropriate treatment, the deafness persists or alternatively the ear appears to be completely normal, then the cause is almost certainly neural deafness.

Treatment will naturally depend on the underlying cause.

Wax

There are few things quite as satisfying as syringing out a pair of ears blocked by wax. In goes the stream of water, out comes a brown oily glob, the deafness is miraculously cured and the pristine earhole looks clean enough to dine off. A Canadian physician, Dr Maurice Ernst, has described how patients can treat themselves with the help of a plastic ketchup bottle. While on holiday learning to windsurf, some water shifted the wax in his ear so it became "quite uncomfortable with hearing loss". He goes on:

> *This sort of thing spoils one's day and a lot of time is spent opening one's mouth as wide as one can in order to equalise the air pressure on both sides of the drum. On a trip to a local grocery store I saw a yellow refillable ketchup bottle of the plastic squeeze type and this seemed like a possible instrument for the job at hand. With one hand I squeezed the bottle full of warm water about two or three times, several pieces of wax were removed and my hearing returned to normal.*

Catarrh (Glue Ear)

If there is no wax in the ear canal then the other possible explanation for conductive deafness is catarrh in the middle ear that dampens down the transmission of sound. This can be treated with decongestant medicines, but the following simple remedy may also be tried: hold the nose and blow out hard to make the ears pop. This is repeated on several occasions.

Presbyacusis

Presbyacusis, or neural deafness, may adversely affect hearing in three ways. Consonants can be difficult to grasp and though it is possible to hear someone speaking, it can be hard to understand what is being said. There may also be an associated problem of volume control, so sudden changes in sound intensity are experienced as big jumps in noise. Lastly, it can become more difficult to distinguish where sound is coming from, to localise who is speaking in a crowded room and from which direction.

The only possible treatment for presbyacusis is a hearing aid. These are available on the NHS or can be purchased privately.

Tinnitus

My ears whistle and buzz continuously day and night. I can say I am living a wretched life.

Beethoven

Tinnitus is the amplification of the noise that can be induced by placing both hands over the ears. Many people experience it – especially those like Beethoven who have some form of hearing impairment. The precise cause is often difficult to locate and may include anything from a defect in the tiny hairs in the inner ear to loss of the hearing nerve fibres themselves, or even an abnormality in the part of the brain that decodes sounds. Tinnitus, not surprisingly, is difficult to treat. A positive attitude from the doctor is very helpful – not just "you have to learn to live with it", but a proper examination, an explanation and reassurance that it might get better.

The most widely used treatment is maskers, based on the principle first noted by Aristotle: "Buzzing in the ears ceases when a greater sound drives out the lesser." There are two possibilities with masking. Deep masking covers up the tinnitus so the sound can be more acceptable than the tinnitus itself. Partial masking provides a low background noise in quiet environments. This device, which is similar to a hearing aid, has the advantage that when switched off the tinnitus disappears for a short period. Allternatively one can buy a Walkman mini stereo and listen to one's favourite tapes.

Some tinnitus sufferers gain relief from yoga, taking a leaf out of the book of Eastern mystics they seek to exploit the naturally occurring tinnitus created by placing the hands over the ears. The ears are closed by the fingers and attention is focused on the sounds that are heard. With practice the mind is able to hold on to progressively finer and subtler sounds until eventual liberation is reached. An alternative is the yoga exercise known as 'beating the drum': Using the forefingers, close the flaps of each ear and then beat on the nails of the forefingers with the next digit.

Some people find relief from massage, the optimum site being behind the ear lobe and over the depression formed in front of the ears when the mouth is open. Finally some people may be helped by drug therapy. Clonazepam, an anti-epileptic drug, has its advocates and the depressed can be helped with appropriate anti-depressant medication.

Tasting

Our perception of the subtleties of taste and smell decline with age. The two are of course related – as it is everyone's experience that a nasty cold makes even the most appetising of meals appear bland and dull. There is unfortunately little that can be done about taste loss, other than to increase the intensity of the desired sensation – puddings should be made sweeter, potatoes saltier. It seems sensible also to emphasise the non-gustatory aspects of food that make it pleasurable. Hot food should be hot, not lukewarm. Cold drinks should be cold. Efforts should be made to make food look attractive and textures – the slithering avocado, the rawness of al dente vegetables – becomes increasingly important. Some seasonings stimulate the nasal aspects of taste, such as horseradish, ginger, cloves, cinnamon, pepper and pimento. These should be used more frequently in cooking.

Smelling

Complete loss of smell can come on acutely after a cold or other respiratory tract infection. With luck it will improve with time, but sometimes when the smell does return it is a peculiar disagreeable sensation described as 'old wet biscuit'. There are two possible treatments. A ten-day course of steroids can sometimes lead to a temporary improvement and so might be tried in, for example, the run-up to Christmas. Alternatively the drug Theophylline – taken as 250 mg three times a day for up to eighteen weeks – can in some patients permanently restore smell function. This is at least worth a try.

9

MOBILE

We stay mobile by staying active – walking up and down stairs, a brisk walk on an autumn day or, for those inclined to do something more strenuous, a jog around the park twice a week. There is no reason why people should not stay mobile well into their ninth decade and it is a mistake to presume that aches and pains are only to be expected. Modern treatments, both mainstream and alternative, are now so effective, every effort should be made to identify whatever might be reducing one's mobility with a view to putting it right.

Aches and pains are usually due to either 'arthritis' or 'rheumatism' which as they are often, incorrectly, used inter-changeably, need to be defined. Arthritis is an affliction of the joints usually of the wear-and-tear type as in an arthritic hip. Rheumatism, by contrast, refers to inflammatory problems of the muscles and tendons, which are frequently tender and painful on movement. In general it is not difficult to tell what is amiss: a nagging ache in the hips is likely to be wear-and-tear arthritis, a shooting pain down the leg is probably sciatica, while a tender point over the shoulder or elbow with pain on movement is due to inflammation of the tendons or tendonitis. Whatever the precise cause, the approach to treatment follows similar lines, so in discussing how to stay mobile I will first discuss the principles of treatment, before moving on to review the specific conditions that may be responsible.

General Principles of Treatment

The purpose of treatment is to reduce pain and loss of mobility. It might be *medical*, drugs that are either taken orally or injected; *physical*, that is rest and manipulation; or *alternative* techniques employed by osteopaths and chiropractors. Finally, *surgery* may be necessary. Most people start with their family doctor, who provides the medical treatment – straightforward painkillers plus one of the anti-inflammatory drugs. The next step is the physiotherapist at the local hospital, who provides the physical treatment such as heat, massage and gentle manipulation. Those with persisting problems, especially of the back, tend at this stage to take themselves off to an alternative practitioner such as an osteopath or acupuncturist to see what he can offer. Finally, sufferers may need the attention of a specialist rheumatologist, if they have a condition like rheumatoid arthritis, or an orthopaedic surgeon to give them a new joint.

Medical Treatment

The first and simplest treatment is an analgesic, aspirin or paracetamol, alone or in combination with codeine. These can be taken intermittently when needed or, if the pain is persistent, in adequate dosage every four to six hours. Next come the non-steroidal anti-inflammatory drugs (NSAID for short), so-called because they suppress inflammation, though they are not as powerful as steroids. Some of these, like Nurofen, are household names that are considered so safe they can be bought across the counter from the chemist without a prescription. They usually need to be taken only once a day, and are for the most part of equivalent potency. Your doctor will prescribe the one with which he is most familiar, though, and this is important, some patients do seem to do better on one type than another. Hence if they appear to be ineffective, it is well worth trying another.

The drawback of these drugs is that they cause indigestion due to irritation of the lining of the stomach which, if serious, can cause bleeding or even an ulcer. This is obviously a serious limitation, but there are a variety of ways round it. If the site of the pain is localised, then applying the NSAID as a cream to the skin surface allows sufficient to be absorbed for it to work. Another possibility is to take the drug as a suppository, which obviously will not irritate the lining of the stomach. Alternatively, it may be combined with drugs that reduce the amount of acid (such as Cimetidine) or protect the lining of the stomach such as Arthrotec.

One step up from the NSAIDs are steroids. They are very effective when injected directly into a tender spot as in tendonitis or into an inflamed joint. Their well-known side-effects – thinning of the bone, puffiness of the face, diabetes and raised blood pressure – have given them a bad reputation, but such problems only develop in those who have to take them in high doses for long periods.

The standard medical treatment is therefore quite straightforward: a combination of an analgesic and an anti-inflammatory with or without steroids injected locally, or in certain cases taken by mouth. Other valuable medical treatments include cooling sprays and the anti-anxiety drug Diazepam, both of which help reduce muscle spasm.

Physical Treatment

Heat and cold: The local application of heat dilates the arteries under the skin, thus improving the blood supply, and is useful for stiff joints and muscles. By contrast, cold in the form of ice is useful for treating acute conditions such as tendonitis. An ice cube is rubbed back and forth over the tender point, the feeling of cold is followed by a sensation of burning and itching and then there is numbness with the relief of pain.

Massage: Light massage heightens the threshold of the skin's sensory nerve endings, thus decreasing pain and increasing relaxation. When done vigorously it helps loosen the skin, which tends to lose its elasticity over sites of chronic muscle spasm.

Alternative Therapies

Manipulation: Manipulation works best for back problems. It is available in physiotherapy departments at hospitals or from alternative practitioners of the arts of osteopathy and chiropractic. The osteopath tends to put joints through the full range of movements and then a bit further, while the chiropractor relies on short sharp thrusts to reposition joints and overcome muscle spasm.

Acupuncture: Acupuncture is very good for the treatment of chronic pain. The pain nerves running up and down the spinal cord can be inactivated by local nerve fibres acting as a 'gate'. Thus, local stimulation with an acupuncture needle brings down the gate and inhibits the pain.

Diet: Some patients may be much helped by a diet low in animal fats (meat and dairy products), with an increase in polyunsaturated fats (vegetable oils and fish). Some find their arthritis is precipitated by 'trigger' foods like fruit, alcohol or preservatives and improve if these are excluded from their diet. The only way to determine if this might be relevant is to try a series of exclusion diets, removing one item of food at a time from the diet and assessing the effect.

Surgery

Persistent pain due to arthritis of the hips and knees is probably best treated with a joint replacement. These operations are so good and successful that there is little point in prevaricating and waiting for the pain to get worse. Surgery may also sometimes be of value in back pain.

Having reviewed the general principles of treatment, it is now time to consider the specific conditions that may give rise to loss of mobility.

1. Generalised Aches and Pains

Aches and pain 'all over' are invariably a sign of some under-lying illness. They may be the first symptom of the onset of the menopause, an underactive thyroid, Parkinson's disease or the inflammatory condition polymyalgia.

Polymyalgia – a generalised inflammation of the muscles – becomes increasingly common from the age of sixty onwards. Its cause is not known. The onset is often quite sudden. The major complaint is of aches and pains around the shoulders with stiffness of the joints early in the morning – indeed sometimes sufferers can only get out of bed by rolling or being rolled out by their spouse.

There may be tenderness over various joints and a general feeling of ill health. There may be a loss of appetite with a consequent loss of weight and some patients may defer seeking medical attention for fear they might have cancer. Diagnosis is confirmed by doing the ESR blood test (as discussed in Sorting Things Out). Treatment is with steroids, which produce an almost miraculous improvement, although for some the treatment has to be maintained for several years.

2. *Rheumatism*

Tendonitis: When there is a local tender point over a bone with pain on movement of the muscle, then tendonitis – an inflammation of the tendon part of the muscle as it is inserted into the bone – is the likely diagnosis. The classic example is tennis elbow, on the outer aspect of the elbow but it can occur virtually anywhere: at the shoulder, the base of the thumb or the heel. Treatment in each case is the same, with either anti-inflammatory drugs or a steroid injection.

Firbrositis: Fibrositis is the equivalent of tendonitis in muscle. There is usually a trigger point – an irritable focus which when stimulated by stretching or direct pressure, causes pain in the surrounding area. Any muscle can be involved, though it is usually around the shoulder girdle, upper neck or down the back of the leg. Treatment can either be with a cooling spray that reduces the spasm or injection of a local anaesthetic

122

combined with a steroid directly into the trigger point. Acupuncture is much favoured.

Frozen shoulder: Pain and loss of movement of the shoulder joint is known as a frozen shoulder. It is a particularly frustrating condition because it lasts so long – for anything from one to three years – and can be remarkably resistant to treatment. There is usually a spontaneous onset of pain, which increases in severity and is worse at night, followed by limitation of all movements of the shoulder.

In the early acute phase the pain should be controlled by painkillers and exercising of the arm discouraged. Anti-inflammatory drugs, though often prescribed, are not particularly helpful and the best of treatments is early – that is within the first four weeks – direct injection of steroids into the shoulder joint.

After a while the acute pain subsides and the chronic phase begins, with loss of movement as the dominant symptom. Gentle physiotherapy can be introduced at this stage, but if it persists then specialists usually advocate manipulation of the shoulder under a general anaesthetic to improve the mobility of the joint. Some favour a more aggressive approach, as a former consultant at the Royal Orthopaedic Hospital puts it:

Once the acute phase has subsided, manipulation under anaesthesia should be performed and followed by steroid therapy. A few days after manipulation (which often causes a temporary exacerbation of symptoms) intensive physical treatment should be instituted to main a range of movement. This type of management can reduce the period of disability from eighteen months to eighteen weeks.

3. Arthritis

There are many different causes of arthritis, including gout, where uric acid crystals precipitate into the joints, and rheumatoid arthritis, where the tissue surrounding the joint is inflamed and eats away at the cartilage. The commonest form, however, is osteoarthritis, a wear-and-tear phenomenon of the large weight-bearing joints of the hips and knees. In osteoarthritis, the cartilage – the smooth glistening surface over which a joint articulates – becomes cracked and fissured, revealing the bony tissue underneath. To compensate for this, bone grows outward from the side of the joints providing a sort of splint, alleviating the pressure on the joint but increasing its stiffness. The combination of the loss of the cartilage and the splinting mechanism explains the two main symptoms of pain and stiffness, as well as the crackling sound made as the joint moves.

The treatment in the early stages is as already described, with analgesics to control the pain and anti-inflammatory drugs like Nurofen and Indomethacin to dampen down the inflammation and stiffness. If, as sometimes occurs, the joint becomes swollen, then draining the fluid off with a needle while at the same time injecting a small dose of steroids can give temporary relief. Physiotherapy is important, as one of the problems with painful joints is that the muscles surrounding them become weak and wasted due to disuse and these need to be strengthened.

The only curative treatment, however, is a joint replacement, which should be considered sooner rather than later. The longer the operation is postponed, the longer the pain and misery that have to be endured and the more likelihood that some other medical illness may intervene to make the operation more difficult.

Regrettably, the waiting list for these joint replacement operations can be anything up to two years, so although you might be getting on fairly well with drug treatment, your family doctor should be encouraged to refer you early for a consultation with the orthopaedic surgeon. He may advise that an operation can safely be deferred for a year or two, but at least by the time it will prove really useful, you will be at the top of the waiting list.

Hip and knee replacements provide excellent relief from pain and permit ordinary movement, such as walking and climbing stairs, but they will not restore the joint to normal, so activity that involves stressful repetitive movements, such as tennis or jogging, are not advised and exercise has to be sought in other ways, such as bicycling or swimming. One of the problems sometimes encountered is that in the elation of being pain-free, patients put too much strain on their other joints, so that although their new hip or knee feels fine, they rapidly become incapacitated by pain from other joints.

Hip Replacement

The hip replacement operation proceeds as follows: the surgeon makes an incision down the side of the leg and the muscles surrounding the joint are separated. The ball joint at the top of the femur is cut away and replaced by one usually made of cobalt. The socket, or acetabulum, in the pelvis into which the ball joint fits is replaced with a hemispherical shell. The stay in hospital is about ten days. Crutches are necessary for the first six to twelve weeks and then over a period of another month or two the transition is made to normal walking.

The major complication is the, gratefully rare, problem of

infection of the new joint which can be very difficult to treat and may require its removal to permit the infection to be cured, after which a further hip replacement can be inserted.

The results of a hip replacement are described as 'good' or 'excellent' in ninety per cent of cases while a serious complication occurs in about five per cent. In the longer term, there is no doubt the joint does become loose in its socket although usually this doesn't seem to make much difference to mobility. One in ten patients will need a further operation over a ten-year period.

Knee Replacement

Though the benefits of hip replacement are widely appreciated, many doctors are more sceptical about the same operation on the knee. Certainly the knee joint is more complicated and the results of early operations were often less spectacular due to mechanical problems. However, a recent review has found a 'good' or 'excellent' result in ninety per cent, with virtually all being able to walk at least two miles without pain and a similar percentage being able to climb stairs without support. These results are very similar to those with hip replacements and the real problem is not the efficacy of the operation, but the limited number of orthopaedic surgeons with the necessary expertise.

4. Back pain

The onset of back pain usually precipitates the following pattern of events. The sufferer takes painkillers for a few days. These make little difference, so he goes to his doctor who asks him to bend over and touch his toes and advises that rest for a week or two with a prescription for anti-inflammatory drugs will probably improve matters. If it does not, then the sufferer, advised by a friend, takes himself off to an osteopath or chiropractor who is much more enthusiastic, gives him a more detailed examination and does some manipulation. Occasionally the results are dramatic and long lasting, but more often there is temporary improvement and occasionally the pain gets worse. If the latter, it is then back to the family doctor who advises referral to an orthopaedic surgeon, which may mean a long wait. Once seen in hospital, another thorough examination is performed and, except in unusual circumstances where there may be evidence of pressure on a nerve, the patient is referred to a physiotherapist who does further manipulation and advises on exercises. With luck, the back pain will gradually get better, if not the cycle may repeat itself.

Why, the patient might quite rightly ask, can no one tell me exactly what the matter is and how to put it right? Why does there seem to be so much contradictory advice – the doctor advises rest, the osteopath manipulation? One person says you should exercise your back, another you should not aggravate inflammation by so doing.

The simple answer is that it can be very difficult to pinpoint the exact cause of back pain, as the structures involved are so complex. First, there are the spinal vertebrae piled one on top of each other which articulate with each other, through two sets of joints. Then there are the intervertebral discs that separate them, the ligaments linking them together, three sets of muscles running up the side of the spine and nerves that issue from the spinal cord through holes in the vertebrae. Any of these structures may be out of alignment, inflamed, torn, bruised, plucked or pressed and all can cause pain. This in turn explains why recommended treatments are often contradictory and the likelihood of success something of a hit-and-miss affair. Thus, if the vertical joints are out of alignment, manipulation may push them together and the patient will feel better immediately. If, however, it is the ligaments that are bruised, the manipulation may exacerbate this so the patient may wish he had stuck to his doctor's advice of persisting with rest and local treatment.

The two common sites of back pain are in the neck and lower back.

Neck Pain

The main symptoms of neck problems – besides pain and stiffness – are a persistent headache, which starts at the back of the skull and radiates over the top, and is usually attributed to spasm of the muscles of the neck as they connect to the base of the skull. Alternatively, if the nerves are being pinched by a vertebra, then the pain will radiate to the top of the shoulders and down into the arm.

The many forms of treatment include a combination of painkillers, anti-inflammatory drugs and topical cold sprays. It may be necessary to wear a cervical collar for a few weeks to stretch the spaces between the vertebrae and take pressure off both nerves and joints. Alternatively, traction with a sling under the patient's neck attached to a weight behind the head is recommended where there is clear evidence of pressure on the nerves.

If, despite all this, the pain is severe and persistent, a scan may be necessary to see if a nerve is being pressurised which may rarely need to be relieved with an operation.

Low Back Pain

Most cases of low back pain will, as discussed, be difficult to classify. Here, the choice lies between your family doctor's advice of rest and anti-inflammatory drugs with some gentle manipulation from a physiotherapist at the local hospital, or recourse to manipulation which may be combined (but this can only be given by a medically qualified practitioner) with an injection of a steroid and a local anaesthetic.

There are, nonetheless, several better defined types of back pain with more specific treatments:

Prolapsed disc: The disc between the vertebrae may slip to press on a nerve or group of nerves, causing pain to radiate down the back of the leg and into the foot.

The immediate requirement is rest at home, with healthy doses of painkillers and anti-inflammatory drugs. In severe cases it may be necessary to be admitted to hospital for traction, to separate the vertebrae and take the pressure off the nerves. Most episodes get better within four weeks, though some have to stick it out for three months or more.

This type of acute back pain is the sort for which chiropractors, osteopaths and other manipulators claim the greatest success. There is no doubt that in skilled hands a prompt dramatic relocation of the intervertebral disc by manipulation will save the patient weeks of lying on his back.

If, despite these endeavours, the pain persists, then a few may need an operation. A scan or special X-ray will show exactly where the nerve is being pressurised and then, depending on the surgeon's preference, one of a variety of operations is performed.

The results of surgery are not brilliant, but then surgery is

129

only performed on the most difficult cases which have failed to improve with conventional treatment. Patients can expect considerable relief from pain and recovery of mobility, but over the long term over half will still have residual symptoms for several years. This might seem rather difficult to explain; after all, if whatever is pressing on the nerve is removed, one would expect the problem to go away, Often, however, there is more than one process at fault – not just a prolapsed disc but other mechanical problems in the back as well.

This point has a wider significance because it reflects the difference in perception between the patient and surgeon about what needs to be done. The patient wants to be finished with his pain, and seeks the help of the specialist. The surgeon has seen many cases where an operation has produced a series of new problems. It can be very difficult to cope with those in whom pain persists after an operation, so surgeons tend to be very selective about those whom they will operate on, concentrating only on cases where the result is likely to be good.

Nerve entrapment: The nerves running out of the spinal column may also be nipped by a bony prominence of the vertebrae, and not surprisingly this causes the sciatica type of pain similar to that felt with a prolapsed disc. This tends to be unwavering, day and night, and not much helped by changes in position. Sitting is uncomfortable, and driving any distance is impossible.

The conservative approach of painkillers, analgesics and injections of a local anaesthetic is best, though in a fifth of patients some form of operation may be necessary.

Vertebral instability: When the vertebrae move against each other due to laxity of the ligaments running up and down the spine, the result may be chronic backache which is made worse by sudden movement and walking. The best options are exercises to strengthen the muscles of the back and surgery is suitable only for a minority.

5. *Osteoporosis*

The final, potentially very serious, cause of loss of mobility is osteoporosis or thinning of the bones. Osteoporosis is painless and poses no problem until it is complicated by a fracture, especially of the wrist, which occurs when falling on the outstretched hand, or of the vertebrae of the spine or of the hip joint. It is obviously a good idea to prevent osteoporosis and women taking Hormone Replacement Therapy (HRT) can slow down the thinning of the bone quite dramatically. Some doctors believe that regular calcium supplements in the form of three tablets of Sandocal a day may, by strengthening the bone, also be useful.

When a fracture associated with osteoporosis has occurred, then treatment directed at strengthening the bone should be considered in the hope of preventing another one. The drug Etidronate given intermittently significantly increases bone strength and reduces by half the risk of further fractures.

10

CHEERFUL

Melancholy is a necessary and inseparable accompaniment of an old and decrepit person . . . after seventy years all is trouble and sorrow.

> *The Anatomy of Melancholy*, Robert Burton

Luckily times change and two centuries after Robert Burton's observations, seventy-year-olds are no longer 'old and decrepit' and far from all being "trouble and sorrow", most surveys reveal they are happy and content.

Nonetheless, it would be absurd to deny that the sad losses and physical illnesses that occur more frequently from the age of fifty onwards can make it difficult to 'stay cheerful'. In some, gloominess may slip into depression, whose treatment is the subject of this chapter and whose main features have been described as follows:

The person suffering from depression feels (with increasing severity) desperate and suffers from insomnia with early morning waking and anxiety as well as muscular aches, trembling, sluggishness, nausea, bladder and gut malfunction, headaches, loss of appetite and sex drive, confused thinking and so on. This profound feeling differs little from

133

*that felt, say, in severe influenza. The main difference, how-
ever, is that the 'flu patient will be back to normal in a
few days whereas the depressed patient may start off opti-
mistically enough: "I feel ill now and unable to cope but tomorrow I'll feel better," but tomorrow arrives and he feels
slightly worse. He learns that his optimism of the previous
day was unjustified.*

The main symptoms of depression – cheerlessness, misery and
loss of pleasure in life – may seem indistinguishable from the
gloominess that accompanies bereavement or physical illness,
but the distinction is that the mood is out of proportion both in
intensity and duration to the precipitating factor that might
have given rise to it.

The precise way depression may affect an individual will
obviously vary but the two most severe forms are readily
recognised: apathetic and agitated. Those laid low by apathy
will stay at home all day, rarely venturing out, do not read the
newspapers or even bother to watch television. Friends are
ignored because, quite legitimately, the patient may feel he has
nothing of interest to say. This apathy can lead to a state of
virtual immobility, where thought processes become so impaired that there might be suspicion of a serious intellectual
deficit.

In agitated depression, by contrast, there is a stronger
element of anxiety, often focused on the body, producing
a wide range of hypochondriacal symptoms with the con-
tinual worry about the heart or bowels or that a heart attack or
stroke may be imminent. There is, of course, a close relationship between mind and body, so these mental problems *are*
felt physically – agitation is experienced as palpitations of the
heart or a feeling of faintness, while the loss of appetite may

134

produce physical changes in the body, such as loss of weight.

The problem, as always, is to distinguish between those whose complaints are due to agitated depression from those in whom there is an underlying medical cause. And, of course, it does happen that people are told they are suffering from a depression and neurosis only for it to turn out they have something seriously wrong. The distinction between hypochondriacal depression and physical illness may be difficult, but should be possible if the doctor takes a careful history and performs the necessary blood tests and X-rays.

Treatment

Those unfortunate enough to be afflicted by depression require treatment, but first it is necessary to consider possible extraneous or exacerbating factors, of which the commonest is that the mental state may be a side-effect of medication taken for some other condition. Virtually any drug can cause depression, but the main culprits are those used for treating raised blood pressure, such as betablockers, anti-inflammatory drugs like Indomethacin and cholesterol-lowering drugs. Depression may also be a dominant symptom of two illnesses: Parkinson's disease and an underactive thyroid (hypothyroidism). Further, any physical illness such as pain from an arthritic joint or shortness of breath from poorly controlled heart failure can make the sufferer pretty miserable, so it is important to ensure that these have been treated as effectively as possible.

We now turn to the specific treatments for depression, which are of two sorts: psychological or physical (directed to changing the chemistry of the brain) antidepressant drugs and electroconvulsive therapy (ECT).

Psychological Therapy

There are more than enough reasons for feeling depressed – loneliness, bereavement, conflict with children and physical illness, so on the basis of 'a problem shared is a problem halved,' it is always useful to talk with a friend or relative or indeed the family doctor. Sometimes, however, talking may not be enough and some form of psychological therapy may be appropriate, of which much the most effective is Cognitive Therapy. This, as its name implies, is concerned with what, or more precisely how, people think about themselves and the world around them. Thoughts exert a profound influence on feelings and so distorted patterns of thinking (such as the belief that life is pointless) can profoundly affect the emotions. In Cognitive Therapy such distorted patterns of thinking are identified and, in theory, once corrected the feelings they cause – depression and anxiety – should be ameliorated. The key insight of Cognitive Therapy is that one's state of mind may be influenced by 'automatic thoughts' which operate at the margins of consciousness, a sort of continuous internal monologue of which one might hardly be aware. When these automatic thoughts are brought out into the open, examined and discussed, then patients report an enormous improvement in their emotional well-being. Cognitive Therapy looks for the causes and solutions of mental problems, not in long-forgotten events from early childhood, but in patients' everyday lives. Treatment lasts months rather than years and crucially has been consistently shown to be highly effective.

Drugs

Antidepressants: The underlying physical problem in depression is presumed to be – though it is difficult to prove – some abnormality of the chemistry of the brain, particularly of the neurotransmitters such as adrenalin or serotonin, the chemical messengers that transfer the messages from one nerve to another. Drugs that increase or alter the balance of these neurotransmitters have for long played a central role in treatment. There are many different types, but the most widely prescribed are those which increase the level of serotonin, of which the most popular is fluoxetine, better known as Prozac, which is taken as just one pill a day and whose side-effects are less marked. It does not work immediately, but after a fortnight or so, patients frequently report that "the sun has come out" and though they may not have completely rediscovered the joys of living, nonetheless their sense of hopelessness has been alleviated.

Some people naturally are resistent to the very idea of taking antidepressants on the basis either that they are just chemical crutches, or indeed that they may be addictive, but this is to misunderstand their purpose. Their great virtue is to break the vicious cycle of the sense of hopelessness that accompanies depression and by restoring the psyche to near normality, give people the confidence that they can indeed be cheerful again.

Initiating treatment should certainly not be considered lightly, but once decided upon it should be pursued vigorously. A major problem with antidepressant treatment is that the attitude towards it tends to be half-baked. Patients will often tell their doctors that after a few weeks they feel a bit better and so wish to stop. The temptation to do so should be resisted and medication continued for at least six months and, if necessary, longer. If, as sometimes happens, one type of antidepressant is ineffective, then another should be tried.

Tranquillisers: Fearfulness or anxiety may, not surprisingly, be a feature of the agitated depression already described, or indeed of any physical illness, as it is only natural to be apprehensive of what the future might hold. Under the circumstances it may be appropriate to take a minor tranquilliser, of which Lorazepam is probably the most effective. At the very least it will ensure a good night's sleep and, by countering the sense of chronic exhaustion, help the restoration of psychological well-being.

Electro-convulsive therapy: Electro-convulsive therapy, or ECT, is highly effective if much frowned upon nowadays. It is reserved for those who fail to respond to treatment with drugs. A short-acting general anaesthetic is administered and an electric current of low voltage is applied to the base of the brain. Treatment is given twice a week for between a fortnight and six weeks. There can be a transient loss of memory after two or three sessions, which usually improves spontaneously, although it has been suggested that ECT works by erasing the unhappy incidents that precipitated the depression in the first place. ECT is so effective – working in about 80 per cent of those receiving it – that it might well be considered preferable to antidepressants. Its vital role in the treatment of severe depression is summed up by the distinguished psychiatrist Professor Brice Pitt, who has observed "it can be as negligent to withhold ECT as not to remove an obstruction from the windpipe of someone who is suffocating". One of the many thousands who have benefited from ECT put it like this:

The treatment is spaced at precise intervals, two a week, so
I knew that at precisely 10 a.m. on Tuesdays and Thursdays
I would receive a general anaesthetic. From complete con-

sciousness to unconsciousness a period of maybe three seconds elapses when I have the profoundly satisfying experience of escaping from myself and the endless and unbearable feeling of illness. But it is neither this pleasure nor the possible efficacy of a brief spell of unconsciousness that here concerns me; rather the fact that I was having, what was then completely novel, thoughts which were optimistic. As the physical symptoms of my depression lifted I slowly unlearnt the deeply ingrained pessimism of my recent past.

11

SEXY

The essence of the sexual history of the modern male has been wittily summarised by the American writer Gail Sheehy. It starts, after puberty, with a period of *unlimited potency*, moves on to the *trajectory from twenty to forty* culminating in "full sexual mastery", then on to the *faltering fifties* where men find a more 'tender, feeling side that needs to be expressed' and ultimately the *sixties potency crisis*, when a man must "use it or lose it".

There are many reasons, both physical and psychological, why the sex lives of both men and women should become less intense with time, but the belief that this is some way inevitable has been transformed by the wonder drug of the nineties – Viagra. This is the most sophisticated and effective of a group of drugs known as the New Aphrodisiacs which, for those who might wish it, offer the prospect of enjoying a fulfilled sex life well into the sixth decade and longer. It has also refocused attention on the wider aspects of sexuality that are the concern of this chapter.

There are essentially two components of the human sexual response: the libido or sexual desire, which is strongly influenced by the effects of the sex hormones on the brain, and physical performance, the mechanics of the sexual act. They will be considered separately.

141

The Libido: Men

The male sex hormone testosterone, produced primarily by the testes, plays a defining role in the maturation of the sexual organs and from then onwards in the production of sperm. It is not, contrary to common perception, directly involved in the mechanics of sexual intercourse, but rather through its effect on the sexual centres in the brain is responsible for the psychological desire for sex, otherwise known as the libido.

This important distinction is based on observations in men whose sexual problems were found on investigation to be due, for a variety of reasons, to low levels of testosterone in the blood. When this testosterone deficiency is corrected with testosterone supplements, not only do they regain their sexual desire but simultaneously the ability to 'have sex'.

With time, the amount of testosterone in the blood may fall, or alternatively the tissues of the brain may become less sensitive to its effects which has led some, but certainly not all, doctors to infer that the decline in sexual activity with age may be due to a decline in libido that could be restored to normal by taking testosterone supplements. This has been dubbed the male menopause or viropause because of the clear analogy with the much more dramatic fall-off in the levels of the female hormone oestrogen and progesterone, which occurs during the female menopause.

The male menopause, if it exists, is claimed to cause the same sort of symptoms including irritability and loss of sexual desire but these could just as easily be psychological because it is a common experience that stress and overwork can also cause fatigue, irritability and loss of sexual libido. As there is no objective test to show these symptoms are directly related to reduced testosterone levels in the blood, the obvious answer would seem to be to take testosterone supplements and see what happens. Men who have done so, at least anecdotally, report marked improvement in their general well-being and the quality of their sex life.

This still does not prove the existence of the male menopause, as the testosterone supplements might simply be acting as a 'tonic' in the same way that anabolic steroids may improve the performance of athletes. The reason for the current controversy about the male menopause and its treatment is thus obvious. If the decline in testosterone were the genuine cause of loss of libido then it would be 'medically respectable' to treat it, but if the testosterone supplements are just working as a hormonal 'tonic', then a prescription would be ethically just as dubious as prescribing anabolic steroids to athletes.

Some might think "if it works, why not try it?" which is fair enough were it not that testosterone replacement therapy can increase the risk of prostate cancer in the same way that HRT in women can increase the risk of breast cancer.

For the moment, the question of whether the male menopause exists, and if so whether it should be treated, remains unresolved. It would, however, be a fair comment that those in whom problems of sexual performance are primarily due to loss of libido (and there is not an obvious psychological problem such as depression) should consider the possibility of taking testosterone supplements. Meanwhile, the possible increased risk of prostate cancer can be minimised by regular screening tests.

The Libido: Women

The precipitous decline in the female sex hormones during the menopause has clear physical and psychological effects, notably the decline in vaginal secretions and loss of sensitivity of the female sex organs. It can be restored with Hormone Replacement Therapy and is another very good reason why women should take it. Female libido is, however, also influenced by the male sex hormone testosterone. Women who, for a variety of gynaecological reasons, were treated with testosterone, reported marked, sometimes dramatic, increase in their libido. This encouraged some doctors to advise women who, despite being treated with HRT, still have a low libido to take in addition a small dose of testosterone. The suggestion is that the hormone increases the susceptibility to sexual stimulation, heightens the sensitivity of the external genitalia and the intensity of sexual gratification. A limiting factor is, however, that the dose of testosterone has to be fairly small to avoid the masculinising side-effects of a deep voice and the growth of facial hair, which is why there is less than unanimity amongst doctors over whether this treatment is as beneficial as some claim.

Physical Performance: Men

The hydraulic mechanics that initiate and sustain an erection are so reliable it is impossible to imagine that they might falter – but they do and with increasing frequency from the fifth decade onwards. This is not surprising, as the erection depends on a subtle interaction of nerves and blood vessels both of which become less efficient with time. The initial stimulus arises from nerves in the penis that dilate the arteries in the corpora spongiosa – the three columns of tissue running along the shaft. The blood flow increases, so do their volume, until a full erection is attained. Inevitably, then, the slowing of the conduction of nervous impulses and narrowing of the arteries will impair this process, causing either impotence or difficulty in maintaining an erection once it is achieved. The underlying problem is clearly physical, but failure, or more often fear of failure, can make matters worse. Indeed, one of the most interesting findings of the New Aphrodisiacs to be discussed is that some men find the self-confidence gained from their successful use cures this psychological source of impotence. The dearth of treatment for age-related impotence in males of the past has been replaced by something of a cornucopia of options. Before discussing them, however, it is necessary to emphasise how frequently medication for other conditions can cause impotence as a side-effect. The commonest offenders are two drugs widely used for the treatment of blood pressure – Bendrofluazide and betablockers such as Propranolol. The list also includes the anti-ulcer drug Cimetidine, Maxolon and virtually any of the drugs used for the treatment of depression. It has been estimated that these drug-related causes of impotence are responsible for 25 per cent of male sexual problems and every effort should be made to change to some other form of medication without side-effects.

It is time now to turn to specific forms of treatment.

Drugs

Viagra works by prolonging the action of a chemical called nitric oxide that is involved in the dilation of the arteries. It is effective in two-thirds of patients, though can cause headaches, flushing and dyspepsia. It is, with a few exceptions, not available on the National Health Service, but can be obtained on private prescription from the family doctor. Viagra has rather eclipsed the other New Aphrodisiacs mainly because of its efficacy and because it is so easy to take. Nonetheless, those in whom it does not work should consider the possibility of the other options which include the drug Muse, which has to be instilled directly into the urethra; Caverjet, which has to be injected directly into the penis; and Yohimbine, an ancient African aphrodisiac that is also available on private prescription.

Some older men whose erectile potency is unimpaired nonetheless find their sexual relationships compromised by premature ejaculation. This, too, may have a physical cause and often improves with a small dose of the antidepressant Amitriptyline, one of whose side-effects is to delay orgasm.

Mechanical

For those who do not like the idea of taking drugs, there is the alternative option of using a vacuum constricting device which works by pulling blood into the penis by vacuum and then maintaining tumescence by applying a rubber ring at the base of the phallus (this is also a useful tip for anyone with difficulty in maintaining an erection). The cost of the apparatus is considerable, but there is no restriction on the number of times it can be used.

Physical Performance: Women

In women, a lack of sexual responsiveness may be due to loss of elasticity and lubrication of the vaginal tissues associated with the decline of oestrogen levels at the menopause. The treatment is HRT or the local application of oestrogen cream. It has also been suggested that Viagra also markedly increases the intensity of the female sexual response.

PART 4

BATTLING THE BIG THREE

Three main obstacles stand in the way of getting to ninety: heart disease and strokes (where the blood supply to the heart and brain respectively is interrupted) and the dreaded disease cancer. They are all age-determined, that is, the longer you live the more likely you are to encounter one or other for, as described in the Introduction, in their different ways they involve a breakdown in the two dynamic systems of the body – the circulation of the blood and division of the cells.

In Living Longer we discussed how they might be preventable or, at least, postponable, by a judicious combination of A Sober Life, Screening and Drugs to Prevent Disease. But that is not the end of the matter. It is equally important to know how, if threatened by one or other of these Big Three illnesses, it is possible to do battle and survive.

12

HEART DISEASE

Heart attacks are bad news and though the epidemic that has affected middle-aged men over the last fifty years is (for reasons unknown) in a steep decline, it remains a serious hazard for those the wrong side of sixty, striking suddenly and unexpectedly out of the blue. The underlying problem, as everyone knows, is that the arteries to the heart become narrowed with time with a porridgy substance known as atheroma – a process that is exacerbated in those who smoke or whose cholesterol levels are too high. The narrowing of the arteries reduces the supply of oxygenated blood to the heart muscle, resulting in angina pectoris (literally pain in the chest). Alternatively, a clot may form in the artery, critically reducing the blood supply to the heart muscle, resulting in a heart attack.

The possibilities for preventing this misfortune were considered at length in the first section of this book. Two aspects of A Sober Life – regular exercise and not smoking – may slow the accumulation of atheroma and thus minimise the narrowing of the arteries. Then as described in Screening, those with raised blood pressure and high cholesterol levels can be identified and appropriately treated with a similar effect. Finally there are two 'preventative' drugs – HRT in women and aspirin which prevent the formation of the clot that causes a heart attack.

We now turn our attention to the various treatments to minimise the symptoms of angina and maximise the chances of surviving a heart attack.

Angina Pectoris

They who are afflicted with angina are seized whilst they are walking (more especially if it be uphill and soon after eating) by a most powerful and disagreeable sensation in the chest which seems as if it would extinguish life if it were to increase. But the moment they stand still all this passes.

William Heberden, 1802

William Heberden's 'disagreeable sensation' is variously described as a tightness (as if the chest is being squeezed in a vice) or a heaviness (as if a weight is pressing down on the chest) with a pain which radiates up the left side of the neck and down the left arm. The explanation for these symptoms, as has been noted, is that there is a fixed narrowing of the coronary arteries that limits the blood flow to the heart muscle. What happens is as follows. As soon as we start walking, the amount of blood pushed out by the heart must increase to supply the leg muscles, but this by definition increases the heart muscle's own need for blood. If this need cannot be met because the blood flow is obstructed, the lack of oxygen stimulates pain fibres in the heart muscle which is experienced as angina. Any form of exertion can precipitate an attack of angina though, as Heberden pointed out, so can a heavy meal, because the heart must pump out more blood to the stomach to aid digestion –

or indeed anything that increases the pulse rate, such as an old-fashioned domestic row.

Most angina sufferers soon learn with great accuracy how much they can do before the onset of their anginal pains. Thus, angina that comes on after walking a mile on the flat will be induced by half a mile up a slight gradient, or a quarter of a mile if there is shopping to be carried as well. At the other extreme, when the coronary arteries are severely narrowed, even something as trivial as brushing one's teeth can bring it on.

It is easy to grasp the image of a fixed partial obstruction to blood flow in the arteries of the heart leading to a stable and predictable limitation of exercise. Symptoms can stay this way for years, and as long as the angina is mild or controlled by medical treatment, it is compatible with a near-normal life expectancy. In some the angina improves over time, which is often attributed to the opening up of smaller arteries, thus increasing the amount of blood available to the heart muscle. Alternatively, angina may become unstable, coming on only after minimal exertion or even at rest. Here medical attention should be sought urgently if the complication of a heart attack is to be prevented.

Diagnosis

The diagnosis of angina is usually self-evident. The crushing chest pain is so typical and so well known that the sufferer has usually made the diagnosis before visiting the doctor to have it confirmed. There are, however, as discussed in Sorting Things Out, three situations where anginal pain can be misinterpreted as being due to some other condition. They are:

- if the pain comes on after a meal, it can be attributed to dyspepsia or indigestion
- if the pain in the left arm is the most prominent symptom it may be attributed to 'neuralgia' caused by arthritis in the cervical spine pressing on the nerves that pass down the arm
- if the pain comes on in bed at night, this is sometimes attributed to heartburn, where acid refluxes from the stomach up in to the oesophagus.

Investigation

There are three ways of confirming (or discounting) the diagnosis of angina:

1. *The electrocardiogram (ECG)*: An ECG is the standard test for angina, but it is of limited use because the pain can still be due to angina even if it is normal. Contrariwise, if the ECG is abnormal this does not necessarily mean that angina is the cause of the pain.

2. *An exercise ECG*: The 'exercise' electrocardiogram is much more reliable. ECG electrodes are placed on the chest of the patient, who is then encouraged to walk on a treadmill. A positive diagnosis can then be made by examining the ECG when the anginal pain comes on, which will show changes due to the relative deprivation of oxygen reaching the heart muscle. This obviously distinguishes pain due to angina from that of other causes. If the exercise ECG is normal, the patient can be reassured that whatever else might be going on the heart seems all right. If it is positive, it gives an objective assessment

of how severe the angina is: that is, how easily it is brought on by exertion.

3. *Coronary angiogram*: The next stage after an exercise ECG has confirmed the diagnosis is to X-ray the arteries to the heart (a coronary angiogram) to pinpoint the site of the narrowing and to determine its severity. This is essential if an operation is contemplated either to dilate the blockage or to bypass the narrowing.

In summary, most cases of angina are easily diagnosed by the description of the symptoms. No further investigations are required unless it is thought necessary to confirm or exclude diagnosis in those with an unusual presentation or with chest pain 'of unknown cause', or if the angina is severe enough to justify surgery.

Treatment

Ideally, treatment of angina will abolish the symptoms alto-gether, but usually the most that can be hoped for is to reduce its severity so that an increased amount of exercise can be done before the anginal symptoms supervene. There are two ways of doing this. The first is to dilate the arteries with drugs such as GTN, which increase the amount of blood flowing down the coronary arteries. The second is to reduce the amount of work the heart muscle does when exerted by slowing the pulse rate – usually with drugs called betablockers.

The choice of treatment will depend on the severity of the symptoms. Occasional angina, say once or twice a week, can usually be treated with the occasional tablet of GTN under the tongue. If the angina is worse than this, it is usual to add another drug, such as a betablocker. If the angina is not controlled on this medication, then a decision has to be made whether some form of surgical intervention is required, either dilating the arteries directly with a balloon (coronary angioplasty) or bypassing the obstruction (coronary artery bypass graft).

Surgical treatment

Surgery – whether an angioplasty or a bypass operation – is much the most effective treatment for angina, because it restores the blood flow to the heart muscle, eliminating the symptoms in seven out of ten patients. Further, as will be seen, in some circumstances surgery can prolong life.

The main indication for surgery is angina on minimal exertion such as climbing a short flight of stairs. It could, however, quite reasonably be argued that it should be considered in anyone whose anginal pain seriously compromises their pleasures in life.

The first step is to establish the site and severity of the narrowing and, as already discussed, this involves having a coronary angiogram. Here a thin catheter is introduced into the femoral artery in the groin and manipulated into the aorta until it rests against the heart. The three major coronary arteries – the left main branch, the circumflex and the inferior – are then entered in turn and a dye is injected which demonstrates the site and degree of narrowing. The dye is also flushed into the main cavity of the heart – the left ventricle – so the strength and co-ordination of the contracting heart muscle can be determined. This takes about twenty minutes in skilled hands and the premedication should abolish most of the anxiety associated with the procedure. At the moment of injecting the dye, the doctor will say "you are now going to feel a rather warm sensation in the head" but one patient described it as "a burning sensation in the head, back and rectum of impressive severity".

Having viewed the angiogram the heart specialist will advise one of three possible options:

1. *Do nothing*: If the narrowing of the arteries is too widespread and the functioning of the heart muscle is seriously impaired, the best advice is just to carry on with medical treatment.

2. *Coronary angioplasty*: Here, a metal wire tipped with a balloon is introduced through the femoral artery up into the coronary arteries, the balloon is dilated and the obstruction is flattened like 'a footprint in the snow'. Next, a fine metal tube is left in place to ensure the obstruction does not recur.

3. *Bypass surgery*: This is the third option that the heart specialist may advise and is one of the great triumphs of medicine. The sternum is cut open, revealing the beating heart within the chest. The blood is diverted through a heart-lung machine which takes it out of the heart, oxygenates it and returns it to a vein. The heart is stopped, a vein is removed from the leg, one end is sewn to the major artery emerging from the heart (the aorta), and the other on to the coronary artery past the obstruction. The heart is restarted, the heart-lung machine disconnected and the sternum repaired with metal stitches. The patient is transferred to the intensive care unit for a couple of days and discharged from hospital soon after. A normal life can be resumed after two or three months.

The results of surgery are very impressive: eighty per cent of patients have no angina one year after the operation, and fifty per cent still have no pain ten years later. As the main effect of angina is to limit exertion, patients find that within a month or two they are already much more active than they have been for a long time.

There is also no doubt that in some instances surgery improves the prognosis – that is, it reduces the subsequent risk of having a fatal heart attack. This particularly applies to those whose narrowing is primarily in the left main coronary artery, or who have generalised narrowing of three or more arteries. Here the surgical patients do significantly better than those who are only treated with drugs.

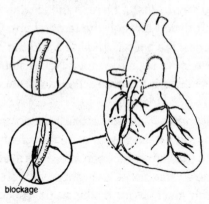

blockage

The coronary artery bypass graft: a vein (taken from the leg) is used to connect the aorta to the coronary artery beyond the site of the blockage so blood can then flow freely to the heart muscle.

Making a decision

In an ideal world, everyone with angina would have a coronary angiogram to determine the degree of narrowing of the coronary arteries and to find the few for whom the simple procedure of coronary angioplasty might be effective and those for whom a bypass operation would, as well as relieving their symptoms, prolong life.

In reality this does not occur, and the option of surgery is essentially restricted to those whose symptoms of angina are poorly controlled by medical treatment. For those over the age of sixty-five, this is probably no bad thing: if they have mild angina, the best advice is to continue with medical treatment. Those with more serious symptoms must be advised by their heart specialist, but in general if the prospect is that of spending the last years of one's life severely disabled by symptoms, then an angiogram proceeding to an operation is probably the best option.

Unstable Angina

When the anginal pain comes on with minimal exertion and unpredictably at rest, this is known as unstable angina. This is a halfway house between chronic stable angina and a full heart attack (to be discussed in the next section), and a medical emergency, as failure to seek prompt medical attention substantially increases the risk of a heart attack.

Most unstable angina is a complication of stable angina, so a patient who for months or a year has found he can walk a mile or two before his pain intervenes suddenly finds this is reduced to a hundred yards or less. Alternatively, unstable angina may be the first indication of coronary heart disease.

The cause is an accumulation of platelets (or blood clotting cells) on the already narrowed coronary arteries, thus narrowing them still further. Treatment therefore requires thinning the blood with aspirin (which antagonises the clotting tendency of platelets) and heparin to prevent the clot from getting any larger.

Unstable angina usually improves with these treatments, at which point a coronary angiogram can then be done to decide whether angioplasty or bypass surgery might be of value. Very occasionally, the symptoms are not controlled by medical treatment and surgery has to be performed as an emergency.

Heart Attack

In a heart attack, a clot or thrombus forms in an already narrowed coronary artery, thus completely obstructing the blood supply to the heart muscle. The victim has a constricting chest pain radiating up to the neck, down the left arm, a feeling that life is being squeezed out, a sensation described as "imminent dissolution". There is naturally the fear that 'this is it,' with much anxiety that something disastrous will happen before medical help arrives.

It is not, however, always like this. There may just be a sense of malaise or discomfort, combined with the refusal to believe that whatever is happening could be serious. A doctor described it like this:

I jumped up from the lunch table and helped my wife carry a new bed upstairs. At the top I had an unpleasant indigestion feeling somewhere between the sternum and the throat; it went almost immediately but returned as I carried the mattress upstairs. The meal at the restaurant the night before had been exotic and it was obviously a mistake to jump around so soon after lunch. It was probably heartburn – milk and sodium bicarbonate produced a satisying burp and gave some relief. Sitting down quietly with a newspaper did not really help but it was difficult to hold the news-

paper up without discomfort in the forearms. How odd; if a patient gave that history I would immediately suspect a myocardial infarct (heart attack) but then I was not a patient. More milk and bicarb. Out to the garden to try chopping wood. Singularly unhelpful. Pity that there were not useful medicines in the house, try lying down for a while. I wonder what to do if it does not go away.

Much better after lying down for twenty minutes but cannot waste an afternoon like this. Walk downstairs. Feel grim again. Walk down the garden to the car to get a book. Try walking faster back up the path. Forced to stop. Good gracious. Did I really have to stop, or was I imagining it?

Am I being neurotic? The pain has been present for nearly four hours so think it is time for some action. Feeling rather foolish tentatively ask wife to get ECG machine from car. While wiring self to ECG fully expecting it to be normal, swear wife to secrecy for fear of mirth of colleagues. Switch on. Trace showing a classic heart attack appears before astonished eyes. Tell wife. We dither about what to do as we are new to the area. Whether to phone the ambulance direct. Wife thinks it will be discourteous to nice new GP. Gentleman to the last, so phone GP. Identify self and problem. GP very helpful and calm. Bad luck, old chap. Arranges everything rapidly.

In the past, the friendly family doctor, as in this instance, would drop round, confirm the diagnosis either from experience or by doing an ECG, prescribe some morphine and advise a few days in bed in the comfort and quiet of the patient's home being looked after by a loving spouse. Then medical fashion changed. The major threat to life following a heart attack is the development of an abnormal rhythm of the heart muscle that can be lethal but is treatable with drugs or an electric shock, so all patients with a heart attack were bundled into an ambulance, taken to the nearest hospital, ensconced in a hospital bed and connected up to a monitor. There they had to recuperate as well as possible in the dreary atmosphere of the coronary care unit, surrounded by patients suffering from the same condition for whom every so often something went badly wrong, the dispiriting effect of which induced gloomy thoughts.

Coronary care units certainly saved a few lives, but did not make a lot of difference, probably because those who were going to die from an abnormal rhythm complicating their heart attack did so in the hour or so after it happened, while those who made it to hospital were the ones who would have survived anyhow. They began to go out of fashion, but what saved them, and has made a trip to hospital almost inescapable, was the discovery in the mid-1980s that the clot in the coronary artery could be dissolved by powerful blood thinning drugs before serious damage to the heart muscle had occurred. These drugs can really only be given in hospital and as, not surprisingly, they have a favourable effect on the outcome, hospital admission for a heart attack is now almost essential.

When a heart attack is suspected the following action should be taken, assuming there is someone present to help:

1. Lay the victim on the floor.
2. Give him an aspirin and, if he takes GTN for angina, one tablet of GTN to dissolve under the tongue.
3. Telephone for the ambulance and then the general practitioner.
4. Hold his hand and try to feel the pulse.
5. If he seems to be 'going off', hit the chest hard three times, pinch the nose and blow into the mouth and repeat.

6. Try to be calm.
7. When the doctor arrives, or the patient reaches casualty, morphine and a drug to stop vomiting are given to control the pain.
8. A needle is inserted in a vein through which the blood-thinning drug streptokinase is infused slowly over one hour. This 'reopens' the artery by dissolving the clot in approximately three-quarters of cases. There is a small risk of bleeding after the infusion, but as the potential benefit is so great, this can effectively be ignored.

When the infusion is finished, the artery is kept open with another blood-thinning drug, heparin, for a couple of days. Then the drip comes down and it is time to get out of bed. Further progress follows a time-honoured fashion: walking to the toilet, then up and down the ward, moving on to a bit of exercise and a flight of stairs followed by home within about ten days.

The combination of aspirin and streptokinase increases the chances of surviving a heart attack from eighty-eight per cent to ninety-two which may not seem a lot, but as heart attacks are very common, it adds up to a lot of 'saved lives' every year.

In the immediate aftermath of a heart attack, the two priorities are to prevent another one and to get fit.

Preventing a recurrence

1. Drugs

- *Betablockers* prevent the risk of a further heart attack by around twenty-five per cent. Treatment should continue for about a year

- *Aspirin* shows 'favourable trends' in reducing the subsequent risk of a heart attack
- The blood-thinning drug *warfarin* after much debate, has now been shown to reduce the risk of a further heart attack by thirty per cent
- There is currently great enthusiasm for also prescribing *cholesterol-lowering drugs*, though these should really be restricted to those in whom the cholesterol is markedly elevated.

Not all people can tolerate these drugs. Betablockers may exacerbate heart failure if it is present; they are harmful for those with bronchitis and can cause general tiredness and loss of energy. Warfarin has to be carefully monitored with regular blood tests. The simplest advice, then, is that everybody should take aspirin and for those who have had a major heart attack the possibility of taking a betablocker with warfarin for a year should be considered if there is no obvious reason not to.

2. Surgery

It would seem sensible following a heart attack to visualise the coronary arteries with a coronary angiogram. The decision can then be made whether to improve the blood flow to the heart muscle with an angioplasty or bypass surgery as already described.

Getting Fit

A stay in hospital, besides providing a safe if perhaps uncongenial haven for recovery, provides an opportunity for meditating on how things are going to be different as soon as the release papers are signed. Resolutions are taken to lead an altogether healthier and essentially more ascetic life, no more late night-dinner parties, no more drinking and eating to excess, certainly no more smoking and lots of regular fresh air and health-giving exercise.

Returning home, there is usually some uncertainty about how vigorously to pursue these new resolutions. It is useful, then, to imagine what is happening to the part of the heart that has been damaged – strong fibres are replacing the dead heart muscle, so in six weeks all that can be seen is a narrow scar, just as follows a cut on the skin.

The first fortnight is therefore best spent pottering around at home, after which an arbitrary rule of thumb would be to walk about half a mile a day and increase this by a further half mile every week, so that by six weeks the regular quota of exercise is about two miles a day. This may have to be modified if you feel you have overdone it.

Some hospitals provide rehabilitation classes for those recovering from a heart attack, under the supervision of a phsysiotherapist. This is certainly not to everybody's taste; the last place one feels like being is inside a hospital again. No one should feel guilty about turning down the offer; there is nothing to suggest formal rehabilitation has any great advantage over 'doing one's own thing'.

Some questions

Driving?
This is allowed after two months, provided it does not cause chest pain. Long journeys should be avoided.

A special diet?
Small, regular meals, especially for those who need to lose weight, is probably the best dietary advice. There is no need to

cut down on fat, but fish a couple of times a week is known to have a small effect in reducing the risk of further heart attacks.

Drink?

Alcohol is good for the heart. Enjoy it, but not to excess.

Sex?

This is deemed safe after six weeks, although it is difficult to know on what basis this advice is given. A GTN tablet taken before intercourse will prevent angina developing as well as maintaining the strength of an erection.

Flying?

Allowed after six weeks, but get someone to carry your bags.

Sport?

Time to give up squash and take up golf.

The future?

This absolutely depends on the severity of the heart attack. Small heart attacks are quite common and indeed may not even be noticed at all – so-called silent heart attacks. Recovery from moderate heart attacks is usually complete, but those who have had a major one involving part of the wall of the left ventricle of the heart are usually disabled to a certain degree from shortness of breath.

In summary, there is no doubt that appropriate action can reduce the severity of a heart attack and indeed save lives. Anyone experiencing chest pains should ensure that they are diagnosed promptly and treated urgently.

13

STROKES

'Stroke', which for the young evokes the imagery of gentle seduction, acquires for those the wrong side of fifty the very different connotation of a sudden and dramatic felling – the stroke of the axe against a tree. The underlying problem, as with heart attacks, is of the sudden interruption of blood flow to the brain – indeed, it has been suggested that a more appropriate term would be a 'brain attack'. The sticky blood cells called platelets form a clot or thrombus in the artery, critically reducing the flow of oxygenated blood to the brain cells which cease to function.

There are in addition two further ways in which the blood flow can be interrupted, which are very relevant to the possibility of preventing strokes. The first is an embolus – a small clump of platelets that has broken away from a heart valve of narrowed artery elsewhere in the body, which then whizzes round the circulation before getting stuck in one or other of the arteries to the brain. Alternatively, one of the blood vessels in the brain may burst, causing blood to haemorrhage into the brain with predictably dire consequences.

Whether the cause of a stroke is a thrombus, embolus or haemorrhage, the nature of the subsequent disability obviously depends on which artery, and so which part of the brain, is involved. If it is the motor cortex, there is loss of movement. If it is the sensory cortex, there is loss of sensation and so on. Some strokes are considerably more serious than others and in order to understand why, it is necessary to appreciate how the nerves in the brain are organised.

They start, as it were, on 'B roads', one bundle serving a single function; these come together to form 'A roads'; and finally merge into 'motorways', transmitting their impulses from the whole of one side of the brain down into the spinal cord.

Self-evidently, a stroke at 'B road' level will only interfere with a localised part of brain function. So if it involves the part of the motor cortex controlling the hand or foot, these will be paralysed. If the frontal lobes are involved, then intellectual foresight and concentration are impaired. Or again, a small stroke at the back of the brain – the cerebellum – leads to a loss of co-ordination, a tendency to stagger to one side when walking and slurred speech.

More seriously, when the stroke involves a 'motorway' then *all* nerves controlling, for example, the muscular movement of one side of the body, will be affected at one fell swoop. The victim is unable to move his arm and leg and the sensory nerves may be similarly affected, with a loss of sensation on the same side. There will be subtler changes as well. The patient may ignore or not recognise the left side of the body and the balance on that side may well be impaired.

The tragedy of a stroke is that a thrombus, embolus or bleed involving a small artery supplying, in anatomical terms, a small part of the brain can have such sudden and devastating consequences. When a similar process occurs in the arteries to the heart – though there is a small risk of sudden death – recovery is usually rapid and ten days later the patient is well on the road to recovery. The brain, however, is such a specialised organ, its functions so complex, that a similar event has much more serious consequences from which recovery may never be complete.

Preventing a Stroke

The effects of a stroke can be so catastrophic that every effort should be made to prevent it in the first place and this will now be considered in relation to the possible underlying causes.

Thrombus or Haemorrhage

Raised blood pressure is much the most serious risk factor for strokes, due either to the formation of a clot (thrombus) or the bursting of a blood vessel (haemorrhage). This can be avoided by dropping in regularly to see your family doctor every two to three years to have your blood pressure measured and, if it is found to be raised, taking appropriate medication.

The additional methods of avoiding these types of strokes, already described in the section Living Longer, are as follows:

A Sober Life

- *Regular exercise* reduces the blood pressure
- *Diet and smoking* Reducing the amount of salt in the diet has no sustainable effect on raised blood pressure, though for the obese losing weight is useful. Stopping smoking will reduce the risk of a stroke by itself and by encouraging more exercise.

Preventive Drugs

Drugs that reduce the blood pressure, as already described, will prevent a stroke. HRT probably also has a protective role, as does aspirin.

Embolus

The second preventable kind of stroke is that due to an embolus, as this is often preceded by a warning 'shot across the bows', where the signs of a stroke develop but last for less than twenty-four hours. This is known as a transient ischaemic attack (TIA): transient because of its short duration; ischaemic because the symptoms are due to interruption of the blood supply to part of the brain; and attack because it comes suddenly and unexpectedly. Those who have a TIA have a one in ten chance of developing a full stroke within a year. Thus this warning shot needs to be taken very seriously, as treatment with blood-thinning tablets or surgery may prevent a full-blown catastrophe.

The symptoms of a TIA will depend on which artery in which part of the brain has been involved. They come on in a matter of seconds and may be repetitive, producing the same symptoms time and again. There may be transient blindness, when the embolus gets stuck in an artery to the retina, or paralysis when it involves an artery to the motor cortex, or loss of balance, vertigo and double vision when an artery to the cerebellum at the back of the brain is involved.

The three possible sources of an embolus include diseased heart valves, the abnormality of heart rhythm known as atrial fibrillation and narrowing of the arteries to the brain due to atheroma. The precise cause can be further identified with investigations such as an echocardiogram, which outlines the shape of the valves in the heart and a special X-ray or carotid angiogram, which demonstrates the degree of obstruction in the arteries to the brain.

The initial treatment requires giving aspirin and another blood-thinning drug, Dypyrimadole, which together reduce the stickiness of the blood. If the TIAs persist, stronger blood-thinning drugs, such as warfarin, may be necessary.

Next it is necessary to do something about the source of the embolus. The diseased valves of the heart may need to be replaced, or if the X-ray has shown evidence of narrowing of the arteries to the brain, then some doctors will recommend an operation to improve the blood flow – a carotid endarterectomy – where the artery is opened up and the atheroma scraped away. This might seem logical, but it is necessary to be careful as the operation itself may precipitate a devastating stroke. There is, to put it bluntly, a substantial difference of opinion about the merits of this operation, but it would seem that those who have a severe if not total narrowing of the arteries to the brain are likely to benefit.

Treating a Stroke

Despite these preventive measures, strokes still happen and I now turn to considering how they are diagnosed and the various approaches to treatment and rehabilitation.

Strokes are usually painless and loss of consciousness (if it occurs) is of short duration. It may be difficult initially for bystanders to know what is going on, especially if the patient is confused and (if the stroke affects the right side) unable to talk. Peter Medawar, the distinguished scientist and Nobel prizewinner, noticed his first symptoms when reading at a service at Exeter cathedral:

> As I read the lesson I became aware that something was going wrong; my speech became slow and rather slurred and I felt as if I was somehow being dragged down to my left side. Jean [his wife] realised I was having a stroke. She turned to the cathedral dignitary sitting next to her and said, 'My husband is having a stroke, I must go to him.' He tried to reassure her, 'Don't be concerned, dear lady, it is probably the acoustics.'

Sooner or later it becomes clear what is going on and the stroke victim is transferred to hospital, where examination will reveal what part of the brain is affected and the severity of the disability will be assessed. The examination will reveal one or more of the following fundings:

1. *Paralysis* of part or the whole of one side of the body.
2. *Altered sensation* There may be a generalised numbness or alteration of touch perception.
3. *Visual disturbance* The nerves as they pass from the eye to the visual cortex at the back of the brain may be damaged, resulting in a loss of half the field of vision in both eyes on the side of the stroke.
4. *Speech disturbance* There are two types of speech disturbance. The first, as described by Peter Medawar, is a slurring due to loss of control over the muscles that control movement of the tongue. This is called dysarthria (difficulty in talking). Much more distressing is the loss of ability to find the right word for the simplest objects or to make sense of what is being said. This indicates disruption of the speech

centre on the left side of the brain. One victim describes it as follows:

> I could not speak although my tongue worked perfectly well and I knew what I wanted to say. I could not understand what people said to me, though I was not in the slightest bit deaf. I could not read although I could see the words quite clearly on the page; they just had no meaning. As with my speech I knew what I wanted to write but could not find the words, and even then I could not spell.

5. *Loss of co-ordination* Some stroke victims, though not paralysed, are nonetheless severely disabled because they have lost the ability to co-ordinate the several movements necessary to carry out routine tasks. Each movement involved in making a cup of tea, heating the water, taking off the top of the pot, adding the tea and so on, can be done separately, but not sequentially one after the other. This is called apraxia.

6. *Ignoring the affected side of the body, or 'sensory inattention'* This is one of the more bizarre and debilitating consequences of a stroke, as described by Oliver Sachs in 'The Case of Mrs S' in his famous collection *The Man Who Mistook His Wife for a Hat*:

> *She sometimes complains the nurses have not put coffee on her tray. When they say, 'But Mrs S it is right there on the left,' she seems not to understand what they are saying and does not look to the left side. If her head is gently turned so the coffee comes into her sight in the preserved right half of her visual field, she says 'Oh there it is then. It wasn't there before.' Knowing this intellectually she has worked out strategies for dealing with her imper-*

ception. She cannot look left directly, she cannot turn left, so what she does is to turn right – and right again through a circle. Thus she requested and was given a rotating wheelchair. And now when she can't find something which she knows should be there, she swivels to the right through a circle until it comes into view. She finds this similarly successful if she can't find her coffee. If her portion seems too small she will swivel to the right keeping her eyes to the right until her previously missed half now comes into view. She will eat this, or rather half of this, and feel less hungry than before.

The terrible problem with sensory inattention, as can be imagined, is that when the patient ignores the paralysed side of the body, then learning to walk or to use a paralysed arm becomes impossible.

So, though paralysis seems the most obvious disability under which the stroke patient labours, other defects can be much worse. To be sure, the stroke patient is not thrilled at being unable to move his arm or leg, but this can seem trivial compared to the inability to react to the world around, to see, interpret and communicate sensibly with others.

Immediate Treatment

The doctor's examination should elicit where in the brain the stroke has occurred and how severe it is. It will also identify possible predisposing factors like raised blood pressure or a source of embolus from the heart that will later need to be investigated and treated. The precise cause of the stroke – whether it is a thrombus, embolus or haemorrhage – can be determined by doing a CT scan of the brain, but this is not essential, as the immediate management of virtually all patients is the same.

Relatives of a stroke victim can easily be frustrated because so little seems to be being done as, with such a major catastrophe, there really should be some treatment to limit the damage and help recovery. It is not for want of trying, but unfortunately dramatic medical measures at this stage (and quite unlike the situation with heart attacks) have usually turned out to compound the damage rather than relieve it.

There have been many attempts to limit the initial damage to the brain by giving steroids to reduce the swelling of the brain, or even by removing a pint or two of blood to dilute out the blood cells. The general opinion seems to be that they make little difference, though they have their advocates and probably do no harm.

When the stroke is caused by a thrombus or embolus, one might imagine that blood-thinning drugs, as used in heart attacks, might be of value. Regrettably, however, they carry the risk of making things worse by inducing bleeding into the brain. Essentially, dramatic medical intervention at this stage is rarely indicated, other than to give aspirin which, though it will not improve the immediate symptoms, will, by reducing the clotting tendency of the blood, reduce the chances of having a further stroke.

There are two exceptions to this general rule. The first is when there is a 'stuttering stroke' or 'stroke in evolution,' where over a period of twenty-four hours the degree of paralysis seems to be getting progressively worse. Here, blood-thinning drugs may indeed be indicated. The second exception is when the leakage of blood from a haemorrhage may critically increase the pressure within the skull. Here, in certain circumstances, an operation to remove the clot is indicated. A CT brain scan is performed and a neurosurgeon's opinion sought.

Recovery

It can be hard for both the stroke patient and his relatives to imagine in the earlier stages that any meaningful recovery will ever happen – where only a few days before, there were millions of live nerve cells enthusiastically passing neurotransmitter chemicals between each other, providing information from the outside world and sending detailed messages to all of the muscles of the body, now there is just a black hole of dead tissue.

But recovery does occur, the main reason being that a stroke also causes swelling of the adjoining brain tissue, further impairing its function. Once the swelling starts to subside, these functions return to normal. There are three other mechanisms involved in recovery:

- The part of the brain that has been damaged may be taken over by other nerve cells. This remarkable adaptive phenomenon is known as 'plasticity'
- Some damaged nerves may be able to regenerate or regrow
- Rehabilitation – the process of learning ways of coping with, or getting round, apparently insurmountable obstacles – can markedly speed recovery.

The Principles of Rehabilitation

The serious business of rehabilitation starts a few days after the patient has been admitted to hospital. Here, three therapies are particularly important:

Physiotherapy

The physiotherapist can teach the patient how to use his paralysed limbs and thus get him walking again. Two 'hidden problems' in particular have to be overcome – spasticity and loss of sensory feedback.

First, *spasticity*. The muscles of the paralysed limb may appear to be incapable of movement but paradoxically they are in a state of constant contraction stimulated by nerves arising from the spinal cord. To explain. A stroke 'takes out' the dominant nerves from the brain, but leaves the rest of the nerves in the spinal cord intact. Thus, though the main function of the nerves in the motor cortex of the brain is to control the movement of an arm or a leg, they also act to modify or dampen down the reflex action of the nerves at this lower level in the spinal cord – as demonstrated every time a doctor taps the knee, which kicks out instead of making a small gentle movement.

All the main muscle groups act in oppositional balance, where one lot is responsible for extending the knee, another for flexing it and so on. The extensor muscles require greater strength and so are stronger and will, in the absence of the central modifying effect of the motor cortex, override the flexors and as a result the knee will move into a position of permanent extension.

The point of this rather laboured explanation is to emphasise that spasticity (where the spinal reflexes are dominant) must be minimised, so several times a day each affected limb has to be put through its full range of movement to keep the muscle supple. Then, when the paralysed limb is resting, it has to be placed in a position that counteracts the stronger group of muscles. So, the neck must be kept as straight as possible, the shoulders and arms raised, helped by placing them on a pillow, the wrist and fingers straightened (often helped by a splint), the knees must be bent and the foot kept in a position of upward flexion.

The second problem, *loss of sensory feedback*, is fairly obvious if one thinks about it. The co-ordinated movement of a limb is not just a matter of voluntary control of the contraction of muscles, but requires the constant sensory feedback from the affected limb, telling the brain, from second to second, where the foot is in relation to the floor, what particular position the arm is in as it moves through an arc, and so on. It is crucial then to sensitise the limb, so it knows what it is doing at any one time.

Speech therapy

There are, as has already been pointed out, two types of speech difficulty associated with a stroke. In the first, there is a difficulty of articulation due to loss of control over the muscles of speech. The second is aphasia where there is difficulty in finding the right words and stringing them together, which is usually due to a stroke involving the speech area on the left side of the brain. The former responds well to speech therapy, while the latter is much more intractable. It is the frustration of being unable to remember a name or word magnified a millionfold.

Occupational therapy

Occupational therapists can reteach a thousand trivial aspects of everyday life that it is necessary, though incredibly tedious, to have to learn all over again: how to boil a kettle, make the toast, brush your teeth, get dressed and shave.

A Rehabilitation Unit

There is no doubt that following a major stroke the best place to be is on the general medical ward of a major hospital, where the doctors and nurses can keep a watchful eye. After a while, however, the stroke patient may begin to feel he has been forgotten. New patients with more urgent medical problems have arrived on the ward and there is a feeling that the doctor's interest in recovery is not adequately focused.

This is the time to move to the rehabilitation unit which is attached to most hospitals. These may not have quite the excitement and bustle of a general medical ward but they maximise the chance of subsequent independence. The Medical Director of the Foundation Medical Centre in California provides an excellent description of how they work:

Your first impression of the Centre is likely to be unfavourable. It is filled with disabled persons just like yourself. There are lots of other people with strokes. It is all rather appalling. You dislike the enforced intimacy. You hate the wheelchair which with malevolent perversity zigzags around in the corridor instead of proceeding directly forwards.

Your right shoulder constantly aches from the drag downwards from the hand which has no intrinsic movement and is puffy and tender. Instead of using heat on your shoulder they startle you by using a cold compress. At first you shiver with apprehension but then you learn to appreciate the anodyne and anti-spastic qualities of cold.

Meanwhile the leg is doing very well indeed. The rubber shock cord from calf to toe helps keep the toe upward and outward. Soon you graduate from the parallel bars to independent walking in the gym.

The key person in your life is the speech therapist who, by treating you like an equal rather than someone from a foreign country with only partially intelligent speech, helps mend your shattered ego. The sessions are fatiguing, more so than any kind of learning with which you can ever remember being faced. Some days you feel no progress at all is being made. At first numbers were the only things you found easy and the one real pleasurable activity was playing gin rummy. Gradually reading clears up and it is a shock when they tell you to begin learning left-handed writing. This is a slow business.

The occupational therapist teaches you how to struggle with your clothes and tie your shoelaces with your left hand. Well, you can do it but hate to be forced. With the really fatiguing exercises during the day you find yourself sleeping better at night. You also begin to go home for weekends. The family is both fearful and delighted.

All the other patients, whose intellectual and social strata seem so far from yours, are now for the most part, close friends and fellow pilgrims. You have largely abandoned both your fantasies of miraculous, total recovery as well as your gloomy preoccupation. It seems incredible that all this could have happened when at last you are discharged a short eight weeks since the day of the stroke.

Prognosis

The degree of damage to the brain tissue will obviously determine how quickly and how well a stroke patient recovers. It is not easy to assess immediately, but it is a reliable rule of thumb that if function returns within the first fortnight, the overall prospect is very good. At the other extreme, unfortunately, there are certain types of disability which are associated with little hope of full recovery, including sensory inattention – the tendency to ignore the affected part of the body – and loss of postural control – the inability to sit or stand.

Recovery usually follows a common pattern. First comes the ability to sit in a chair and eat alone. Then control over the bowel and bladder function returns, then the ability to walk with help and to shave and wash. Next comes the ability to get out of bed and walk alone, proceeding to managing the stairs and finally eating and dressing alone. Most recovery will have occurred within the first three months, but there will still be some, albeit quite slow, further recovery over the next six months.

Going Home

The much anticipated homecoming can be a shock. The stroke patient realises 'this is it' and he fears that the memories of the safety and happiness of home life might be a mirage. For many, things will never be the same again, as nothing can compensate for the loss of true independence. Meanwhile, the spouse, or relative, or carer, faces the prospect of the continuing responsibility of looking after someone on whom they may have depended in the past.

The success of the return home essentially depends on how everyone adjusts to their altered circumstances and above all the psyche of the patient and 'carer', which go through a predictable pattern of emotional changes.

The Patient's Reaction

The stroke patient is initially optimistic, especially in the first flood of recovery, but when this stabilises and the degree of residual disability becomes apparent, it can easily change to anger tinged with frustration. The simplest task seems full of problems just because previously it was done automatically and unthinkingly. The future holds so little promise that depression sets in and the temptation is to give up.

This depression can be very serious. Its cause – the disability – is unalterable yet if it gets a grip, depression constrains further what can be done, which only makes matters worse. The carer begins to think the stroke patient is lazy, constantly complaining with no apparent desire to help himself. This is the 'can't, but won't' syndrome, also characterised by intellectual decline and importuning behaviour. This is a serious problem and there is some evidence to suggest that it can be helped with antidepressant drugs or electroconvulsive therapy (ECT).

It can be very difficult to decide what is a 'normal' depressive reaction to the effect of a stroke and at what point it moves beyond to become an important impediment to recovery. It is not easy to make this distinction, so perhaps it is justifiable to try antidepressant treatment. The fact that depression is held to be a natural reaction to a stroke is not an argument for not treating it.

Antidepressant drugs can also help in the less common but distressing consequences of a stroke, emotionalism, when the patient veers precipitously from laughing to crying though there is no apparent reason for either.

Perhaps the greatest misfortune of a stroke is the psychological changes associated with damage to the brain. Major personality changes are rare, but there is a loss of control, so previously suppressed characteristics become much more obvious. Someone who previously was merely irascible becomes a chronic complainer; stubbornness becomes intractability; the highly strung perpetually fearful and dependent. These emotional difficulties can be very difficult to cope with other than by establishing firm ground rules.

The Family's Reaction

The family too will go through predictable phases, sharing the excitement and optimism in the early days of recovery, but becoming downcast by the lack of progress, or holding on to unreasonable hopes of what can be achieved. The main enemies here are guilt and exhaustion.

Guilt arises from the constant feeling that one could be doing more which, though commendable in many ways, can cause terrible animosity if the stroke patient appears to be doing less than he can to help himself. Exhaustion comes with overwork; then, instead of one invalid there are two – the stroke patient and his carer.

There is a need here to re-create or rebuild the personal life that might, with luck, reinfuse the relationship with reserves of strength – 'free' periods when others share the burden must be clearly demarcated. Despite this, the carer may end up needing medical help, either supportive or with drugs such as antidepressants. These might be seen as chemical crutches, but why not?

The quality of the relationship that preceded the stroke is central to how well the family copes. Here, paradoxically, those who have already grown slightly apart might actually be better off, as caring is often more easily dealt with when reduced to the simplicities of fulfilling an obligation.

These latter comments really only apply to the more severe types of stroke and it is vital to remember that in the vast majority of cases there is much enjoyable life to look forward to. So, to conclude on an optimistic note, here is the account of a sixty-two-year-old Professor of Anatomy:

I woke one morning and turned in bed. In the course of a few minutes an initial heavy but uncharacteristic dizziness was followed by difficulty in speaking, double vision and a marked paralysis of my left arm and leg. There was no loss of consciousness, no headache, no vomiting and no neck stiffness.

By the end of the first day the left-sided paralysis was almost complete but gradually it improved so that five days later some slight movement and flexion of the fingers and elbow was possible.

There was, as is usual in the beginning, a fairly rapid and extensive recovery. Two months after my stroke I was able, for example, to button and unbutton my clothes, to handle a fork when eating – though clumsily and with reduced power – but both tasks needed much more attention and energy than normal. Later, a slow but steady improvement took place. After six months I could walk very well and could use my left arm and hand for most things.

Repeatedly I made the same striking observation – the mental effort needed to move a severely paralysed limb is considerable. It felt as it the muscle was unwilling to contract, as if there was a resistance which could be overcome by strong voluntary effort. Expenditure of this mental energy is very exhausting, a fact of considerable importance.

Passive movements of the affected limbs are desirable to prevent shrinking of the ligaments and muscles. They have, however, another function. In the beginning, I often noted that even with the strongest effort I was unable to make a voluntary movement of a particular joint, but when the full movement had been passively made by the physiotherapist a couple of times I was able to perform it, although with minimal force. Subjectively it was clear that the sensory information provided by the passive movement helped me to 'direct' forceful movements through the proper channel.

For forty years I had used a bow tie almost daily and when I had to tie it for the first time after my stroke it was, as expected, very difficult and I had to make several attempts before succeeding. The precise finger movements were difficult to perform with sufficient strength, speed and co-ordination, but it is quite obvious that the main reason for the failure was something else.

Under normal conditions, the small, delicate movements follow each other in the proper sequence almost automatically and the act of tying had proceeded without much conscious thought. Now I felt as if I had to stop because my fingers did not know the next move. I had the feeling as when one recites a poem or sings a song and gets lost. The only way to start again is from the beginning. It felt as if the delay in the succession of movements interrupted a chain of more or less automatic movements.

I noted I became much more easily tired than previously from mental work even from ordinary conversation and reading newspapers. There was a marked reduction in my powers of concentration which made mental tasks far more demanding than before. Reading a novel did not cause great problems, but it was often quite difficult to focus my concentration to follow the acute arguments, for example, in a scientific paper. In part this seemed to be due to a re-

duced capacity to retain the sense of a sentence long enough to combine it with the meaning of the next one.

So I found that in addition to the objective changes that occur following a stroke, an alteration in a number of functions which are much more difficult to quantify even though very obvious. They are what one might call general defects in the functions of brain: loss of powers of concentration, reduced short-term memory, increased fatigue, reduced initiative, and other phenomena. It may be argued that several of these changes are due to the psychologically depressing effect of having suffered a stroke. This may play a part but close observation has led me to the conviction that much of the reduced mental capacity must be related to the destruction of brain tissue. It is also astonishing how long it takes for these obvious symptoms to improve. So even after ten months when the paralysis is almost fully recovered I was painfully aware that I was not back to normal. Nevertheless it is often amazing to notice the degree to which restitution may take place.

14

CANCER

Many types of cancer have become curable over the last few decades – and even when a cure is not possible, life can be usefully prolonged. Nothing, however, can make cancer a cheerful prospect, and it is useful to analyse the reasons for the disease's fearful reputation. The patient may feel guilt that the cancer is his own fault due to his 'unhealthy lifestyle', but this only applies to smoking-related lung cancer, as with virtually all the others the most important cause is simply 'getting on'. Then there is the understandable fear of pain and discomfort, but again this is not – thanks to powerful painkillers and nerve blocks – the problem that it was in the past. There may be fear of the hazards of treatment. This was more valid in the past when cancer was over-treated with powerful drugs with grievous side-effects, but nowadays such drugs are used much more discriminatingly and their major side-effects of nausea and hair loss are readily controllable.

Cancer is certainly serious and difficult decisions may need to be taken about the best form of treatment; but it is important to emphasise that the fearful implications of diagnosis arise as much from the images and beliefs widely held about the disease as from the disease itself.

Finding Cancer Early

There is no doubt that diagnosing cancer early, before it has had time to spread, increases the chances it will be curable. This requires, firstly, that potentially significant symptoms be acted on promptly and, secondly, that appropriate screening tests be undertaken. Both topics have already been discussed in Living Longer and When Things Go Wrong, but will be summarised here.

Significant Symptoms

Any new symptom, whether it is a cough or dizziness or head-ache or loss of appetite, which persists or gets worse needs to be investigated. The following are particularly important:

- *Constipation or diarrhoea* lasting for more than two weeks in someone who is normally 'regular' may be due to a tumour of the large bowel
- *Persistent hoarseness* may be due to a tumour of the larynx
- *Loss of appetite or indigestion* These are often attrib-uted to inflammation of the stomach but can be caused by a stomach tumour
- *Bleeding from the vagina* – or in women on Hormone Replacement Therapy, bleeding between periods – may be due to a cancer of the uterus.

Screening tests

There are six screening tests which, if undertaken regularly, can catch cancer at a curable stage.

- The lung: an annual chest X-ray for smokers and ex-smokers
- The breast: a mammogram
- The cervix: cervical smear
- The prostate: PSA test
- The bowel: testing the stools for blood and sigmoido-scopy
- The ovary: ultrasound of the ovaries.

The Diagnosis

Screening will detect some cancers, but most are diagnosed in the usual way following the investigation of a patient's symptoms. Thus, if the problem is a cough, the chest X-ray may show a tumour of the lung; if it is a loss of appetite, a stomach X-ray is called for; difficulty in swallowing, an X-ray of the oesophagus and so on. The diagnosis is then confirmed by taking a biopsy to examine any suspicious tissue under a microscope. This is usually done by passing a 'scope' into the relevant organ – down into the airways, or up the back passage, or into the bladder – to take a snip of tissue, or by removing a suspicious lump or gland.

Next, the cancer must be 'staged' to see how far it has spread locally and whether or not it has disseminated elsewhere in the body. The degree of local spread can usually be determined by a CT or MRI scan, while evidence of spread to, say, the liver or bone is obtained with a special radioactive scan or X-ray.

The staging of the cancer is obviously crucial in deciding how best to proceed. Bluntly, the more limited the cancer appears to be, the more justified are attempts with drugs or surgery to destroy it completely. If, on the other hand, scans or

X-rays reveal the cancer has already spread, then a more conservative approach – limited to controlling the symptoms – is probably the better option.

It is only natural to be apprehensive at the prospect of being put through a complex series of investigations but in reality the methods of diagnosis are quite straightforward: an X-ray of the relevant organ, followed by a scope to take a biopsy, a few blood tests, half an hour in a body scanner and a couple of sessions scanning the bone and liver.

Delay in Making the Diagnosis

Sometimes there appears to have been a delay in making the diagnosis – though this almost always seems to be the case in retrospect. Both patients and doctors may be partially responsible and it is useful to understand why. For patients, the two obvious reasons are anxiety – they fear the worst – and denial – a refusal to face the possibility that their symptoms might be serious. "I was not sure it if was anything", "I just put it off", "I thought everyone had lumps like this" are remarks frequently heard in such circumstances.

These natural responses may subsequently induce guilty feelings of "if only I had gone to the doctor earlier . . ." This, however, is rarely justified, as cancers grow slowly over many years and can spread at any time. Thus, a delay of even two or three months is unlikely materially to alter the outlook.

Alternatively, the doctor might be to blame for the delay. On a busy day, he may prevaricate about doing a thorough examination and ordering the relevant investigations, preferring to say "let's wait and see". To himself he may 'deny' the possibility of cancer, especially in a patient he has known for a long time. Finally, a doctor may suspect (or even know) the diagnosis, but will pretend not to, arguing that the longer the patient remains in ignorance, the less misery he will suffer. Many might disagree with this rather paternalistic attitude, but where the prognosis of the cancer is obviously poor, then ignorance can, for a while, be bliss.

Reacting to the Diagnosis

There are four main ways in which people react to being told they have cancer. The commonest is stoicism: "you can't change what is meant to be". The second is denial where the patient deliberately avoids asking leading questions and seems immune to any hints about what is going on. The third is fighting spirit: "I'm not going to let it get me, I'm going to fight it all the way". Finally, there can be a sense of hopelessness, where the patient becomes preoccupied by his illness, convinced that 'it will soon be over'. It is said, though difficult to prove, that both the 'deniers' and the 'let's fight it all the way' types of response are associated with a better outlook than those whose attitude is either one of stoicism or hopelessness.

Whatever the reaction, everyone feels a mixture of anxiety and depression. The anxiety is usually worse right at the beginning while waiting for the diagnosis to be made and treatment started. Here a mild tranquilliser can be very useful. As for depression, it would be most unnatural not to have some gloomy thoughts but a few are caught in a downward spiral where they start developing physical symptoms like insomnia, loss of appetite and weight, and multiple aches and pains, which can be incorrectly attributed to the cancer itself.

Most people cheer up once treatment has started, if only because their original symptoms – of a cough, or difficulty in swallowing – start to improve. This optimism can sometimes be tempered by the side-effects of treatment which can be very trying, as a surgeon who developed Hodgkin's Disease of the lymph glands has observed:

It is easy to say "enjoy every minute of the day", but when you are suffering from a major illness with its often associated minor ailments and then add in radiotherapy or drugs, there are times when enjoyment is just not possible. At these times it is sufficient not to give in to despair, but to try to adapt one's strength and energy to becoming more resilient and so help the return to the healing phase.

The ability to enjoy each day is, in part, a function of how you organise your life. If you are in some physical discomfort then a day spent chasing around can be agony; on the other hand, if you spend that day at home in comfort, you are able to make running repairs and you can probably turn that day into a plus day, i.e. one worth living. I score each day a plus or a minus and with the adjustment in my pattern and attitude to life, minus days are few and far between.

Some patients, perhaps paradoxically become most depressed only once the treatment is over and the tedious regular journeys to and from hospital are no longer necessary. The reason would seem to be that the period when others took the strain of difficult decisions is over. Rather, the patient is now 'on his own' again with his disease, or the fear that it will recur. The same surgeon already quoted captures this well:

Despite the difficulties I have encountered in the previous nine months, the last month of treatment was the most stressful of my life. During my treatment I was released from expectations placed upon me by myself and close friends. But once it ended and convalescence had begun, the boundaries between what I was doing and what I felt I should be doing became blurred. I reacted anxiously to the realisation that everything around me, including my personal relationships, were in a state of flux. Resentment and anger which I might have dealt with before were expressed with full force afterwards.

Coping with Others

The undoubted difficulties of coping with cancer are not helped by doctors and relations, whose help and support can, for the independent minded, be very irritating. Doctors can be limited by lack of imagination, so they find it difficult to see the world through the eyes of their patients. It is sensible, however, before getting upset by their sometimes offhand or imperious manner to appreciate how difficult 'honest' communication can be. Patients may believe or convince themselves they want to know everything that is going on and may resent the vague answers they receive. The doctor may well see things differently: "This patient is asking all these questions, but does he really want to know the answers?" It is not always easy to tell. Further, the idea that there are necessarily clear answers to all questions is obviously an illusion. No matter how experienced a specialist may be, he is not a soothsayer and thus cannot predict what course the illness will take or what the side-effects of treatment might be.

There are many variations on this theme. The best thing is not to expect too much, and not to be overly distressed by the patently false jolly optimism that sometimes prevails: "There is no need to look so glum, it's a lovely day"; or "everybody's a bit upset when they come into hospital, but you'll soon get used to it". This sort of gratuitous banality could well be done without, but it happens and it is best to ignore it.

Relatives pose a different challenge. They will try to be supportive and encouraging, and want to share the burden. They may even feel guilty about the past, exaggerating memories of indifference and often want the future to be rosier than it is likely to be. It is sensible in these circumstances to insist on personal space or privacy. Thanks, whether gushing or self-denigrating ('you really don't need to bother to do all this'), should be avoided.

Treatment

There are three ways of treating cancer: cutting the tumour out with surgery, destroying the cancer cells with X-rays (radiotherapy), or killing the cancer cells with chemotherapy ('chemo'). The indications for their use will be considered in some detail, but it is appropriate first to make some general observations.

The purpose of treatment is either to 'cure', that is to eliminate the cancer altogether, or to 'palliate', that is suppress the symptoms either at the site of the cancer or to wherever it might have spread such as the bone or liver. The choice of treatment is determined by the stage and the degree to which it has, or has not, already spread. Curative treatments will obviously need to be more radical or aggressive than the palliative. Thus, a small cancer of the lung will first be removed by surgery, after which radiotherapy is deployed to sterilise the area around it and finally chemo will hopefully kill any cells that may already have spread. By contrast, if the tumour is more advanced, then treatment will be limited to radiotherapy alone, which by shrinking the size of the cancer will improve the symptoms it is causing.

There has been much concern in recent years that doctors may be too aggressive in their treatment, seeking to obtain a cure when the realistic prospects of doing so are very slim. The patient then suffers twice – from the cancer which persists despite all efforts, and from the debilitating side-effects of treatment. Patients caught in this unfortunate situation feel quite rightfully resentful and the phrase "I just wish they had left me alone" is often heard.

There are two circumstances in which this happens more frequently than it should. The first is where a major operation like opening up the chest or the abdomen is undertaken, only to find the tumour has spread too far for it to be removed. It might be the surgeon really could not tell until he did the operation that this was the case, but with the remarkable clarity now achieved with X-rays, and in particular with the CT body scanner, it should be possible to tell the extent of the tumour with great accuracy.

The second instance of over-treatment is with chemotherapy. This is now much less likely than in the past, but we should understand how it can happen. Some patients whose initial treatment appears to have been successful may subsequently relapse, which can only mean that their cancer had already spread elsewhere, albeit only a few clusters of cells. Theoretically, then, everyone should be given chemo in the hope of knocking out these undetectable rogue cancer cells. This approach is known as adjuvant chemo, because it is being given in addition to the standard treatment. The trouble is that though chemo can cure several cancers especially in the younger age group, it is much less effective in the much commoner cancers such as those of the lung, breast, stomach and so on, because here the cancer cells are less sensitive to the drugs. As at the time the adjuvant therapy is being given it is not possible to know either whether the microscopic cancer cells have spread or whether they are sensitive to the drugs being given, then, by definition, two groups of patients will be over-treated. The first are those in whom the cancer has already been cured by the initial treatment (and in whom, therefore, the chemo is un-necessary) and those whose cancers have already spread, but which are not sensitive to the drugs – and so the chemo is pointless. This matter will be considered further.

It is appropriate, before considering the three main types of treatment in detail, to mention those circumstances in which it is probably best to do nothing. The immediate and natural response to a diagnosis of cancer is to do something radical to get rid of it. There are, however, three situations in which this may not be the best course. First, there are some small and very slow-growing cancers – notably of the prostate in older men – that may be best left alone. Clearly there is a temptation to do something to get rid of them (it is after all a cancer and so 'better out than in') but in fact if nothing is done and the symptoms are treated if and when they occur, then the outlook is just as good. Similarly when a tumour is discovered acci-dentally, say on a routine chest X-ray, and is too large to be removed but is not causing any symptoms, the likelihood is that it is growing very slowly and any treatment would only make the patient feel worse without changing the outlook. It is sensible, then, to defer treatment until symptoms do develop. Finally, if the tumour is widespread and the patient weak and ill, treatment for the sake of it is fairly pointless. This can be very difficult to accept and often the best thing is to give 'something' – perhaps a short course of radiotherapy – so both patient and, perhaps more importantly, the relatives do not feel they are being neglected.

Surgery

Surgery is the obvious and definitive way of getting rid of a cancer. It is psychologically reassuring to feel the body can be rid of this unwanted growth and surgical operations of some form have been the standard treatment for many years.

There are two reasons, one good and one bad, why surgery is now less popular than in the past. The good reason is that better treatments have been found, in particular radiotherapy, which can, by killing the cancer cells, cure a tumour while simultaneously sparing the patient the surgeon's knife.

The bad, or rather gloomy, reason why surgery is now less popular is that it is increasingly recognised that by the time the cancer is diagnosed, it may already have spread elsewhere. There is obviously little point in having a major operation, if the trouble is just going to crop up again fairly soon.

Surgery may, however, be curative and can often palliate:

- *Curative*: When a cancer is localised to one site and has not spread, then the best method is to effect a cure by removing it in its entirety
- *Palliative*: When the tumour is causing symptoms that cannot be easily treated by other means, then a palliative operation may be necessary. Thus a tumour of the bowel can cause an obstruction, which though incurable, can be bypassed with a colostomy.

197

Radiotherapy

Radiotherapy uses high energy X-rays to kill cancer cells by damaging the genetic material within them. Its great virtue is that it is a very straightforward form of treatment, though it can be daunting to be placed in the middle of a vast machine and bombarded from all sides with X-rays.

There is an initial planning consultation, when the areas to receive the X-rays are marked out on the skin in ink. It is customary to give the treatment in fractionated doses, that is a little bit at a time every day over four to six weeks. The dose and amount of radiotherapy will depend on what is hoped will be achieved with higher or more radical treatment when the intention is to cure cancer. The business of travelling to and from the hospital every day can be tiresome, especially as nowadays the treatment is only done in a few specialised centres, so the distances to be covered may be considerable. Sometimes it may be better to stay in hospital for at least part of the treatment.

Radiotherapy can cure many tumours including those of the oesophagus, larynx, prostate and cervix. Palliative treatment either controls the symptoms of the tumour or may be given just to reduce its size, thus buying extra time before it recurs to cause further problems. Radiotherapy is also very helpful in treating pain from secondary deposits in the bone, for which it is highly effective.

The beneficial effects may not be apparent immediately; in fact it often makes patients feel worse initially as it necessarily kills off not just the cancer cells but normal tissue caught in the 'crossfire'. So the skin over the tumour site may become reddened as with a bad attack of sunburn, or the lining of the oesophagus may become inflamed making swallowing temporarily more painful and so on. Radiotherapy can also cause 'radiation sickness', with tiredness, weakness, nausea and depression. These symptoms are dose dependent, so are only particularly marked in those undergoing a lot of treatment.

They require a certain stoicism and resilience and it is important that the side-effects be countered with appropriate treatment. Thus, the tranquilliser Lorazepam will reduce anxiety, the anti-sickness drug Ondansetron will markedly reduce nausea, Codeine phosphate is invaluable for diarrhoea, while bland ointments and gentian violet help the painful skin reaction.

Radiotherapy treatment proceeds with almost conveyor-belt efficiency, which can prove to be rather dispiriting. The patient sits in the waiting room with dozens of others, the treatment is given and then it is out of the door again. The opportunity to discuss matters may be limited and it would seem sensible to drop in on the family doctor from time to time to discuss how things are going.

Chemotherapy

Chemotherapy, or chemo, is much the most important breakthrough in the treatment of cancer over the last fifty years. Once it had been demonstrated that previously lethal cancers such as leukaemia and lymphoma and others could be cured by a combination of powerful cell-killing drugs, the question naturally arose as to whether the same principles could be applied to the much commoner cancers – the so-called solid tumours, because they arise from solid organs such as the breast, lung, gut and so on. These are, however, biologically very different from the curable cancers, such as leukaemia, as they are strongly age-determined – that is they become much more frequent with each passing decade while the cancer cells, as already mentioned, are much less sensitive to the anti-cancer drugs. The value, or otherwise, of chemo in these cancers has been much debated and so it is useful to summarise its various indications:

- *Curative chemo*: Chemo is a very effective treatment for cancers arising from the blood, such as leukaemia and lymphoma, but can also be curative in some cases of the solid tumours, noticeably those of the lung and ovaries.
- *Adjuvant chemo*: This is in addition to other forms of cancer treatment and has three main applications. It may be used before surgery to shrink the size of a tumour so that it then becomes operable, or in the aftermath to kill off any cancer cells that may have been left behind. The major use of adjuvant chemo, however, as already described, is in the hope of eradicating the small clusters of cancer cells that may already have spread elsewhere, although are undetectable at the time of initial treatment. This certainly, as already mentioned, results in over-treatment, but would seem to be most useful in some cancers of the breast, lung and large bowel where it can increase the long-term survival rate by around ten per cent.
- *Palliative chemo*: This is the third use of chemo, in the same way as surgery or radiotherapy, to improve the symptoms by, for example, making a cancer smaller or relieving an obstruction in, for example, one of the lobes of the lung. If a tumour clearly is 'sensitive', i.e. responds to the drugs, then several courses of palliative treatment can be given.

The major drawback of chemo has always been the serious side-effects of nausea, vomiting, hair loss, diarrhoea and so on. Probably the most important advance in recent years has been the ability to control these side-effects by making treatment more tolerable, therefore increasing the number of people who could benefit from it.

Further aspects of treatment

It is not just the cancer but all the other associated symptoms that may warrant treatment.

- *Tiredness and poor appetite*: These call for a general tonic of which much the best is the steroid Prednisolone. Steroids have a natural euphoriant effect, they cheer people up, improve their sense of well-being and their appetite and thus prevent weight loss.
- *Nausea*: There are now several powerful anti-sickness drugs including Maxolon and, particularly effective in cancer treatment, Ondansetron.
- *Constipation*: The combination of painkilling drugs, poor appetite and general inactivity makes constipation a common problem, which should be treated vigorously.
- *Insomnia*: Many patients with cancer have difficulty in sleeping, which is particularly unfortunate as a good night's sleep does wonders to restore morale. Here a dose of a sleeping pill like Temazepam can be particularly useful, giving a good eight hours' sleep.
- *Anxiety and depression*: Anxiety and depression, as already discussed, are common reactions and are best treated respectively with tranquillisers such as Lorazepam and antidepressants such as Prozac.

- *Pain*: The perception of pain is profoundly influenced by mood and as cancer patients can understandably at times be a bit gloomy, then mood-enhancing drugs as well as analgesics may be necessary. Analgesics come in graded strengths, starting with aspirin and paracetamol, running up through the same drugs combined with something stronger such as codeine all the way up to morphine.

  Morphine is often perceived as a drug of last resort but it can also very usefully be taken as an interim measure before symptoms are controlled by other means, such as radiotherapy. It is best taken in the form of a tablet which, depending on the severity of the pain, needs to be taken twice a day. The drawback, as with all strong painkilling treatments, is that it slows the movement of the gut, thus rapidly inducing constipation. Hence it should always be taken with some form of laxative.

  Certain types of pain do not respond to analgesics and require a different approach. If muscle spasm is present, then this can be relieved by valium. The short stabbing neuralgic pains are helped by drugs commonly used in the treatment of epilepsy. Radiotherapy, as has already been noted, can dramatically relieve pain arising from the bones.

  In the few where pain is not relieved by these means, it may be necessary to be referred to a pain clinic whose specialists deploy a variety of techniques, such as freezing the nerves with a local anaesthetic.

Complementary Medicine

Most practitioners of complementary medicine would not claim that their remedies are in any way effective against cancer, but rather are useful in a supportive capacity. Here two points are relevant – one favourable, the second less so. In their favour complementary therapies do give patients back a sense of control over their lives and their illness. Despite the remarkable advances in the mainstream treatment of cancer it does tend to turn people into passive recipients of toxic treatments in rather depressing surroundings. The attraction of complementary therapy is that it allows patients to take control and fight the cancer from their own resources. Further, the physical treatments that alternative medicines offer, such as acupuncture and aromatherapy, are physically very relaxing and certainly make people feel better.

The negative aspect of alternative treatment concerns an obsession with diet and particularly the promotion of the so-called 'healthy diet' – low in animal fats and high in fibre. There is no evidence at all that what one eats has any influence on cancer; indeed, the alleged 'healthy' diet may even be harmful. Thus, high fat foods such as meat and dairy products have rich tastes and textures and it seems perverse to deny people such pleasures for no good reason. They are also high in calories and so are particularly useful in helping to maintain a steady weight. Further, the supposedly 'healthier' foods, with high roughage content like bread and pasta, increase the activity of the bowel, often leading to flatulence, abdominal pain and diarrhoea. If there is any disadvantage in health terms from alternative treatment, it is that this 'healthy diet' debilitates patients so they are distressed by their bowel symptoms and lose weight more rapidly than they would otherwise.

The 'Best' Treatment

It is only natural to wonder whether surgery, radiotherapy or chemotherapy, as chosen by your specialist, is the best available. Here it is important to recognise that in most situations cancer treatment is well standardised and the question of what should be done is decided by the size of the tumour, the severity of the symptoms and its stage. Certainly some hospitals may be trying out experimental new therapies, but there should be little fear that one is missing out.

It is important, however, to recognise that in certain situations there is definitely a trade off, where the alternative to a radical operation with a high chance of complete cure is a less aggressive operation, or radiotherapy which has a lower cure rate but is associated with a better quality of life. Thus, a tumour of the larynx may be curable with a radical operation, but only at the risk of losing one's speech. Radiotherapy, which preserves speech, is also curative, but in a slightly smaller percentage of patients. Some might think this preferable.

After treatment

So the cancer has been diagnosed, treatment given, some form of guarded prognosis arrived at – what now? There are two images here with which most readers will be acquainted.

Firstly, the treatment seems to have made no difference. It all seems a charade, a waste of time; there is even a suspicion that it made matters worse. In some it can lead to a rapid deterioration. There is reassuringly, however, another scenario which goes like this: "They diagnosed cancer, how long ago is it now, about five years? He went through a pretty sticky time and had to have a couple of operations, even had a colostomy for a while, but you would never know it. He's as busy as ever now. Wonderful really, isn't it, what they can do nowadays?'

When the treatment is over, the specialist will keep an eye on you at a clinic every month or so, and as the next appointment gets further away, confidence grows.

Conclusions

There is no doubting the seriousness of the threat to a long and enjoyable life posed by heart attacks, strokes and cancer and the military metaphor of battling these illnesses is entirely appropriate. And just as military success depends as much on knowing and understanding the enemy as effective weaponry, so it is as helpful to understand the nature of these illnesses as the rationale of treatment.

The challenges posed by the Big Three are very diverse but there are certain unifying themes that are worth emphasising. First, modern medicine is a highly sophisticated enterprise both in its ability to diagnose the cause of symptoms and in treating them so one should expect a clear explanation of what is wrong and how it should be put right. Second, doctors have much to do and are not necessarily the best of communicators. It is always sensible to prepare for a medical consultation by focusing on the most important questions you want answered. They are also, like everyone else, very receptive to expressions of thanks and not surprisingly will often make that extra effort for grateful patients. Finally, modern medicine may be effective but it cannot work miracles. It would be wonderful to have better treatments with fewer side-effects, but for the moment these are not available. It is a natural instinct to wish to try anything if there is even the smallest chance it will be of help.

INDEX

Index